SIEGEL

GALEN ON SENSE PERCEPTION

GALEN ON SENSE PERCEPTION

HIS DOCTRINES, OBSERVATIONS AND EXPERIMENTS
ON VISION, HEARING, SMELL,
TASTE, TOUCH AND PAIN,
AND THEIR HISTORICAL SOURCES

RUDOLPH E. SIEGEL, M.D.

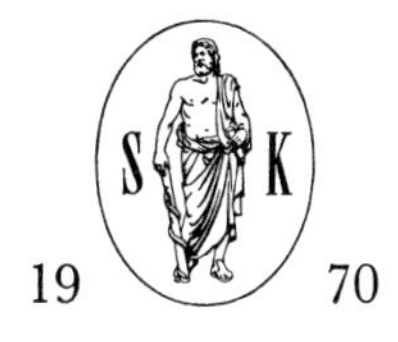

19 70

BASEL SWITZERLAND S. KARGER NEW YORK

Second Part of

GALEN'S SYSTEM OF PHYSIOLOGY AND MEDICINE

(The first part was published in 1968. See Preface, p. 1)

S. Karger AG, Arnold-Böcklin-Strasse 25, 4000 Basel 11 (Switzerland)

Printed in Switzerland by Buchdruckerei Effingerhof AG, Brugg

TO DEBORAH AND ERNEST

CONTENTS

INDEX OF ILLUSTRATIONS

ACKNOWLEDGMENTS

This work was made possible by a grant of the Department of Health, Education and Welfare, and the National Library of Medicine for which I want to express my gratitude. (No. 50-940-A and 1-R01-LM-00011-01, -02 and -03.)

The drawings in the text were made by Mr. M. DIETRICK of the Department of Illustration of the Medical School of the State University of New York at Buffalo. I want to express my sincere thanks to Mr. DIETRICK for his courtesy and great efforts.

I further want to express my thanks for assistance to the personel of the National Library of Medicine, of the Health-Sciences Library of the State University of New York at Buffalo, especially to Mr. ERICH MEYERHOFF, and to many others. I also want to thank Professor PH. DELACY of the Department of Classical Studies at the University of Pennsylvania in Philadelphia for his advice in many questions about translation, especially in the chapter on the visual doctrine of the atomistic philosophers.

R. E. SIEGEL, M.D.
458 West Delavan Avenue, Buffalo, N.Y., 14213, USA

'Il est essentiel de replacer les œuvres étudiées dans leur milieu intellectuel et spirituel, de les interpréter en fonction des habitudes mentales, des préférences et des aversions de leurs auteurs.'

Alexandre Koyre

Isis, *57:* 161 (1966).

PREFACE

The present study presents an analysis of Galen's concepts on sense perception. Half of the book is devoted to the problems of vision for which Galen used a twofold approach: a physiological analysis (if this expression is permitted) based on the pneumatic concept; and a geometrical interpretation, derived from the application of optics and perspective. The difficulty of reconciling these two methods resulted in a compromise which pointed the way for further research. The second part of this study is divided, in almost equal parts, between the problems of perception of sound, odors, taste, touch and pain.

This treatise is a continuation of my systematic analysis of Galen's medical and physiological doctrines, observations and experiments. The previous book was devoted to the problems of blood flow, respiration, humors and internal diseases in Galen's treatises. It also presented, besides a survey of Galen's life and works, a comprehensive list of text-editions, translations and literature on Galen [1].

Only a very brief summary of Galen's basic concepts and their historical sources is given as introduction (p. 3–5) to this study for the benefit of those readers who did not have the possibility to consult my earlier detailed analysis of *Galen's System of Physiology and Medicine* [1].

Each chapter of the present treatise on Galen's doctrine of sense perception includes a discussion of the doctrines of the earlier Greek philosophers on sense perception, since a renewed study of the Greek texts resulted in many instances in an interpretation different from the accepted opinion, especially about vision. The historical survey revealed that Galen's doctrine on sense perception was not a break with the past but an evolution of an old tradition.

As was the previous book, the present work is based on the Greek

1 SIEGEL, R. E.: *Galen's System of Physiology and Medicine; An Analysis of his Doctrines and Observations on Blood Flow, Respiration, Humors and Internal Diseases* (S. Karger, Basel/New York 1968). A continuation of this study is in progress, mainly concerning Galen's concepts and observations in the fields of neurology, psychiatry and the integration of biological functions by the nervous system.

text of Galen's treatises, published by KUEHN [2]. For the Galenic works preserved only in the Arabic language the English or German translations were used.

The quotations from Galen are my own translation from the Greek text of the KUEHN edition [2]. It is indicated when other translations were used.

Square brackets [– – –] in the quotations indicate interpretation by the author of this book, round (– – –) brackets are used to indicate Greek or Latin words or explanatory terms.

Two photographs of drawings of the structure of the eye and ear were reproduced with the permission of the original publishers, W. B. Saunders Co., Philadelphia (Fig. 4 and 9).

2 *C. Galeni opera omnia*, edited by D. C. G. KUEHN (Cnobloch, Leipzig 1821–1833), 22 volumes (modern reprint obtainable).

INTRODUCTION: GALEN'S BASIC CONCEPTS

Galen based his entire system of medicine on three fundamental ideas: his concepts of blood flow, of qualities and of the four humors. The first chapter of the previously published book[1] analyzed the problems of blood flow; the second chapter related the process of respiration and combustion to the concept of qualities; both chapters were dealing extensively with the question of pneuma (spirit). The third and largest chapter was devoted to an analysis of the humors and a description of 'internal' diseases, to use a modern term which actually should not be applied to ancient treatises.

Galen believed that the blood was manufactured in the liver from ingested food; that it then proceeded slowly through both venae cavae to the peripheral organs of the body, carrying the nutrients. A small amount of the venous blood, however, was thought to flow through the right atrium into the right ventricle of the heart. Galen believed that this blood flowed then from the right, the venous chamber of the heart, in two ways to the left, the arterial chamber[1]. He described, for the first time in medical history, that blood could pass through the pulmonary artery (Galen's vena arteriosa) via assumed vascular anastomoses into the branches of the pulmonary vein (Galen's arteria venosa) which leads to the left atrium and ventricle. During this passage the blood became enriched by absorption from the inhaled air of a vital factor, the quality of heat, which entered the blood during its transit through the invisible anastomoses. The other course of the venous blood was supposed to lead from the right ventricle directly into the left ventricle through hypothetical pores of the interventricular septum. This part of the blood was thought to become mixed with the aerated blood arriving from the lungs. On the basis of the Greek text, it could be ascertained that Galen did indeed describe the pulmonary pathway of the

1 SIEGEL, R. E., *Galen's System of Physiology and Medicine* (Karger, Basel 1968); SIEGEL, R. E., Am. J. Cardiol. *10:* 738–745 (1962); also SIEGEL, R. E., Sudh. Arch. *46:* 311–332 (1962). In both instances the text is supported by revised diagrammatic drawings of the blood flow in man according to Galen and to modern concept, of the blood flow in the fetus and in fish.

blood, a fact already acknowledged repeatedly by WILLIAM HARVEY in the treatise *De motu cordis* [1].

Galen, however, assumed that only a few drops of blood entered the left heart from the pulmonary vein with each respiratory cycle. We, therefore, should not speak of a blood flow through the pulmonary vessels or lesser circulation, but of a slow transit of blood through assumed anastomoses of these vessels. The use of the term circulation presumes a coordination between the amounts passing through both pulmonary and peripheral vessels and also indicates a return flow.

Galen described the process which we call arterialization of blood as the formation of *vital pneuma (spiritus vitalis, pneuma zotikon)* in the blood. He also believed that the blood became hot in the left ventricle of the heart where 'combustion' was stimulated by the heat of the vital spirit and the inhaled air. Both the vital pneuma and the heat were then carried by the arteries from the left heart into the entire body. But in Galen's system of blood flow the arterial and the venous blood were flowing slowly toward the periphery to be completely utilized. Needless to say, Galen also described the portal blood flow between bowel, liver and spleen as essential for the resorption of food, the formation of blood, and maintenance and growth of the body.

Galen wrote that, in the arteries entering the brain, the vital spirit was transformed into the *cerebral spirit (pneuma psychikon, animal spirit)* which represented the active principle of the central nervous system. It is important to point out that Galen regarded this spirit also as the active agent of all sensory organs. The principal seat of the cerebral pneuma was believed to be in the ventricles of the brain. But some of this pneuma seemed to diffuse even into the brain matter itself. Generated from the anterior parts of the brain this pneuma was then slowly eliminated to the outside via the third and fourth ventricles and the sutures of the skull. Additional cerebral pneuma was supposedly furnished by air entering the anterior ventricles directly from the nose along the olfactory nerves. This inconsistency—one of the many in Galen's system—had interesting empirical reasons which will be discussed in this study.

The second chapter of the earlier book was devoted to an analysis of the concept of qualities and to Galen's doctrine of respiration. Both ideas were intimately connected since Galen, following the Aristotelian concept of matter, stipulated that all substances were characterized by various invisible (material) qualities. Galen thought that the quality of heat, the most important quality for the maintenance of life, entered the blood during its pulmonary passage. Earlier, Galen had discovered that all blood vessels of the body contained blood, since there was never free air visible in the arterial blood as other physicians had believed. He, therefore, considered as the only acceptable mechanism of respiration that the invisible quality of the vital heat entered the blood in the lung from where it was carried along through the pulmonary veins into the left heart.

It is of utmost importance for our understanding of Galen's system of sense physiology to appreciate that his concept of qualities was also the basis of his doctrine of respiration, of metabolism *(alloiosis)* and of the activity of the brain, and therefore, of course, also of sense perception. The present study will refer, wherever necessary, to these concepts. But a detailed repetition of this extensive discussion could not be included in this study.

A large section of the previous book was devoted to an analysis of the humors and their relation to Galen's concept of disease. The greater part of this chapter, about half of the book, contained a description of internal diseases in Galen's treatises. However, only a general knowledge of these humoral concepts appears of importance for our understanding Galen's doctrine of sensation, since the present study is more concerned with the problems of perception than with disease.

The present work tries to relate Galen's writings on sense perception to the doctrines of his predecessors, to his own philosophical and physiological ideas, and last but not least, to his amazingly detailed anatomical knowledge of the sense organs, especially of the eye. The reasons for Galen's errors will also be explained, since they reveal his scientific method. The added bibliography covers only the present study, since the first book contained a more complete bibliography on Galen and a survey of Galen's writings, including translations into modern languages.

THE CRANIAL NERVES

(See table on p. 9)

Galen's doctrine of sense perception can be better understood, when his account of the anatomy of the cranial nerves has been discussed. Galen wrote that the cranial nerves should be examined on apes, since human material was not available. Apes with rounded faces seemed to him most desirable but difficult to prepare.

> 'The dissection is best made on apes, and amongst the apes in such a one as has a face rounded to the greatest extent possible amongst apes. For these apes with rounded face are most like human beings.'[1]

In the second line, he recommended to dissect the brain of pigs or goats

> 'to avoid seeing the unpleasing expression of the ape when it is being dissected'[2].

Galen refused to follow strictly the anatomical description of earlier anatomy books, since he thought that progress could only be achieved by independent examination of the natural structures. We read in the ninth book of Galen's treatise *On anatomical procedures* which has reached us only in an Arabic translation:

> 'MARINUS has concluded that there are seven pairs, whereas HEROPHILIUS says there are more than seven cranial nerves . . . Whoever does not know this . . . is like a seaman who navigates out of a book. Thus, he reads books on anatomy, but he omits inspecting with his own eyes in an animal body the several things about which he is reading,'[3]

1 DUCKWORTH, p. 10 (1962).
2 DUCKWORTH, p. 15 (1962).
3 DUCKWORTH, p. 10 (1962).

Galen's critical attitude to the traditional teaching methods of his contemporaries evidently did not influence that of medieval scientists who regarded Galen's and HIPPOCRATES' writings as immutable truth.

Galen designated the cranial nerves by only seven numbers, different from those used today. Although he considered some statements of his predecessors as erroneous, he wanted to comply with the contemporary terminology. The authors on whose work he mainly relied were MARINUS, who lived in Alexandria during the first part of the second century A.D.[4], and HEROPHILUS (325–280 B.C.). Galen did not give any other denomination to the cranial nerves but numbers, with exception of the optic nerve.

The first nerve of modern nomenclature is the *olfactory*. Galen did not consider this structure as a specific nerve but as a bulbous protrusion of the brain (see chapter on smell, p. 140), especially since in animals it was much bulkier than a regular nerve. The *optic* nerve, therefore, represents Galen's *first* cranial nerve. Then followed as *second* nerve the *oculomotor* nerve of modern terminology, which moves the eyeball in all directions. The *trochlear* nerve, which rotates the eyeball, escaped Galen's attention. Galen's *third* cranial nerve is called today the *trigeminal* nerve. This nerve is composed of a larger anterior sensory and a smaller posterior motor part which Galen correctly distinguished. According to his observations, motor nerves were harder than sensory fibers. In contrast to our usage, Galen gave therefore a separate number to the motor fibers of the third nerve, enumerating them as the *fourth* cranial nerve.

We call Galen's *fifth* nerve the *acoustic* nerve. Galen did not commit MARINUS' error of considering the facial and auditory nerves as a single nerve, although both leave the brain closely together. But Galen also described a motor part of his fifth nerve, which we designate separately as the facial nerve. He wrote that after its parting from the acoustic nerve it took a longer course through the petrous bone and, therefore, constituted indeed another nerve[5]. He further stated that the sensory

4 SARTON, p. 39 (1954).

5 According to anatomists prior to Galen, especially MARINUS, this motor nerve (facial nerve, modern term) entered a 'blind opening' in the skull; but Galen discovered that this nerve entered a true canal which opened at the lower side of the temporal bone near the processus styloideus (called today canalis Falloppii). Galen stated that this nerve passed first through this bony canal near the acoustic organ in the petrous bone, but that, after leaving this canal, it supplied the motor fibers for the movement of muscles in cheeks, eyelids and forehead (DAREMBERG, vol. 1, p. 589; KUEHN, vol. 3, p. 723; Galen, *De usu partium*, book 9, chap. 10).

part of the fifth nerve penetrated the solid temporal bone (the so-called petrous bone). The ancients had already chosen this name because of the exceeding hardness of the structure of this bone. Galen knew that the 'acoustic' nerve (modern term), representing the larger parts of Galen's fifth nerve, terminated in the auditory organ of the inner ear. He was not aware, however, that the fifth nerve sends two branches into the inner ear, a smaller one to the vestibular organ (modern terminology), maintaining the equilibrium of the body; and a larger one to the cochlea, the auditory nerve in the stricter sense.

Galen considered likewise the *glossopharyngeal*, *vagal* and *accessory* nerves as one single nerve, representing the *sixth* nerve, since they left the skull through the same opening. But he specified:

> 'Neither [pair] consists of a single nerve springing from either side of the brain . . . But each one of the pairs consists of three nerves which come off from three roots.' [6]

The last, the *hypoglossus* nerve, was numbered as the *seventh*. Galen described its course through the lateral foramina of the upper cervical vertebrae [6], but did not visualize all its anastomoses with other nerves.

Further anatomical details will be given in the respective chapters on sense perception.

6 Duckworth, p. 10 (1962).

CRANIAL NERVES[7]

	Modern nomenclature	Galen's notation
I	Olfactory nerve	not defined as nerve
II	Optic nerve	1st pair: optic nerve
III	Oculomotor nerve	2nd pair: no name given
IV	Trochlear nerve	unknown to Galen
V	Trigeminal nerve (motor and sensory fibers)	3rd pair: sensory part 4th pair: motor part of same nerve[8]
VI	Abducent nerve	not clearly defined
VII	Facial nerve	not separated from the acoustic or fifth nerve
VIII	Acoustic and vestibular	5th pair: acoustic nerve (facial nerve not clearly separated)
IX X XI	Glossopharyngeal nerve Vagus nerve Spinal accessory nerve	6th pair: composed of the three, no name given
XII	Hypoglossal nerve	7th pair: no name given

7 Details in DUCKWORTH, p. 8ff.; SINGER, p. 251 (1956); DAREMBERG, vol. 1, p. 583ff. Also GOSS (1966) who translated Galen's treatise on the nerve (KUEHN, vol. 2, pp. 831–854).

8 SINGER's statement, p. 251 (1956), is erroneous; the abducent nerve of the horse, ox or man is too far from the second nerve (Galen's number) to be considered as part of it. GOSS, Am. J. Anat. *118:* 327ff. (1966) includes the *plexus caroticus sympathici* in Galen's fourth nerves. His translation of Galen's text gives ample details. See also DUCKWORTH, p. 195ff.

I. GALEN'S ANALYSIS OF VISION: PHYSIOLOGICAL AND GEOMETRICAL INTERPRETATION AND HISTORICAL BACKGROUND

'Even if I have omitted many things, still this treatise is complete. I did not fail to mention the function of any part of the eye, especially because each part has not only one but a number of purposes.'
(Concluding sentence of Galen's treatise on the function of the eye, Kuehn, vol. 3, p. 838.)

A. THE GEOMETRICAL AND PHYSIOLOGICAL CONCEPT OF VISION

In his treatise *On the function of the parts of the body*[1], Galen (129–200 A.D.) presented a detailed anatomical description of the structures of the eye and surrounding tissues and a functional analysis of the process of vision. One part of his physiological discussion is based on the doctrine of the pneuma, the invisible agent of neural and cerebral activity. The second part deals with the application of the rules of optics and perspective to the understanding of vision. Galen concluded the first part of the chapter on visual perception with the following words:

> 'We have now spoken about almost every aspect concerning the eye, except one single matter, which indeed I would rather not describe at all, so that neither the difficulty of explanation nor its length may cause me to be hated. For in connection with these matters I must touch upon geometrical theory ... As, however, a dream came to me and complained that I had badly conducted myself against the most divine of the organs and had even committed an outrage ... by leaving a work unexplained which so plainly exhibited the highest wisdom and providence for living things, I was obliged to take up a subject which until then I had completely neglected, and to give it some attention.'[2]

1 Galen, *De usu partium:* KUEHN, vol. 3, pp. 759–841.

2 KUEHN, vol. 3, p. 812. Taken from SHASTID's translation with minor changes (p. 8611).

In other words, Galen reminded his readers that the pneumatic explanation of vision gave an incomplete analysis unless supplemented by a discussion of the geometrical aspect of the problem. The recognition of the dual approach by a separate study of the optical and physiological aspect of vision outlined the problem correctly for later research, although we hardly know whether Galen's writings about these questions were known to the later scientists engaged in the advancement of this science.

It may be of interest to follow the last quotation with one of KEPLER (1571–1630) who was the first to understand correctly the physics of the optical media of the eye:

> 'I am going to bring forward not my own observations on the eye but an account combining those published by the most outstanding medical men . . . For then they will scarcely grudge yielding place to me in mathematics in so far as I may be properly well regarded by expert judgement.' [3]
>
> 'Compare the true mechanism of vision as given by me with that given by PLATER, and you will see that this famous man is no further from the truth than is consonant with being a medical man who has not studied mathematics.' [4]

These passages reflect indeed Galen's idea that there were two complementary approaches to the study of vision: the physiological or pneumatic interpretation of the process of vision and the geometrical analysis of both the path of the image to the eye and through the media of the eye. For centuries, neglect of the proper anatomical relationships led, however, to serious errors in the mathematical analysis of vision. Thus, VESALIUS still described the position of the lens as in the middle of the human eyeball, although Galen had known that it was closer to the cornea than to the posterior wall of the eyeball [5]. Even KEPLER based his calculations on an assumed spherical shape of the lens, disregarding that its flattened appearance had already been known in antiquity [6]. KEPLER was, however, the first to come close to a correct

3 CROMBIE, *Kepler*, p. 145. See also CROMBIE (1967).

4 CROMBIE, *Kepler*, p. 139.

5 There are certain differences in lower animals: see DUKE-ELDER, vol. 1, p. 353 ff. In both ox and man the lens is quite close to the cornea. Galen only stated that he dissected ox eyes.

6 CROMBIE, *Kepler*, p. 141; also CROMBIE (1967).

concept of the true nature of the visual process, since he combined the newly acquired knowledge of optical lenses and the camera obscura with a more correct interpretation of retinal function[6].

Neither Galen nor his contemporaries had been familiar with the laws of refraction by lenses[7]. They did not even apply the known laws of refraction to the analysis of the path of light rays through the eye, although they knew approximately the angle at which light rays were deflected when passing from air into a medium of different density. Galen, however, tried to combine the knowledge of a rectilinear propagation of light rays and perspective, as far as they were known, with the results of anatomical studies of the eye and with his doctrine of nerve activity.

In spite of a rather extensive interest among scientists of late antiquity and the Middle Ages, no other comprehensive attempt was made before ALHAZEN[8] to improve the traditional doctrine of vision which was still based on Galen's concepts of anatomy, geometry and the pneumatic doctrine. ALHAZEN (literally IBN-AL-HAITHAM), who was born in 965 A.D. in Basra and died probably in 1038, wrote a treatise *Opticae Thesaurus* which was first printed in Basel (1572). It is commonly accepted that the modern science of physiological optics started with the work of ALHAZEN. He stated:

> 'The treatment of the "what" of light belongs to the natural sciences, but the treatment of the "how" of radiation of light requires the mathematical sciences . . . and the same for transparent bodies into which the light enters.'[9]

ALHAZEN based the attempt to combine optics, mathematics and physiology partly on knowledge of Galen's work. This connection proves the direct influence of Galen on modern optical studies. However, no adequate modern study of Galen's doctrines and experiments on visual perception has been published.

Galen's treatise on vision remained incomplete, since he did not

7 A third century convex lens of 10 diopters of the time of the Ptolemies was discovered, but remained a rare, isolated finding (MAYER, 1946).

8 MEYERHOF (1920) discussed the work of many other Arabic scientists in reference to these problems. GARRISON (1929) dated ALHAZEN's birth at 996 A.D. METTLER and CASTIGLIONI, in their historical textbooks, cited the date as 965 A.D.

9 SHASTID, p. 8702 (1911); see also figure 8 (p. 115).

want to present the geometrical aspect of the problem in all the details known to him and necessary for a thorough study of the visual process. He wrote in defense of this omission:

> 'These sciences make the experts therein hated and unacceptable even to the majority of educated persons.' [10]

These words are a testimony to the difficulties which Galen encountered during his public lectures in Rome. They prove that reference to the optical science prior to and contemporary with Galen is needed. Indeed it is impossible to understand Galen's doctrine of vision without surveying briefly the doctrines of visual perception of his predecessors. Therefore, a renewed study of the visual doctrine of the earlier Greek philosophers was undertaken. This led to an interpretation of their ideas somewhat different from those commonly held. The importance of these sources had become obvious when reading Galen's own biographical treatises and his critical discussion of the opinions of the other philosophers. Furthermore, we find in Galen's writings on vision references to the optical treatises of EUCLID (323–285 B.C.) and we can also demonstrate considerable similarities between Galen's ideas and those of his contemporary, the physicist and astronomer CLAUDIUS PTOLEMAEUS [11]. We may assume that, during or prior to Galen's time, other scientists had published treatises on perspective comparable to those of PTOLEMY. But of the Hellenistic studies on vision only the books of these two authors and of Galen have survived, since most books at the library at Alexandria perished in the holocaust of the Arabic invasion of Egypt (646 A.D.), although it appears likely that the early Christians had burned part of it already in the 3rd century.

At the time of conquest the commander of the Arabic army utilized the scrolls and books of this great library to heat the hundreds of public baths in the city. The victors did not want the books: if they contained opinions which agreed with the teachings of the Koran, the books were

10 KUEHN, vol. 3, p. 812.

11 It appears questionable whether PTOLEMY's name was really CLAUDIUS. The abbreviation for *clarissimus* was *Cl.* The same mistake appears in quotations of Galen's name, whose name was never Claudius Galenus. During the Middle Ages he was called *Clarissimus Galenus*, 'the most famous Galen'. Even the KUEHN edition of his works perpetuated this historical error on the title page.

considered superfluous; if they contradicted the Koran, they seemed to deserve destruction. Thanks to this infallible logic, Galen's treatises remained the only comprehensive medical work of antiquity dealing with visual physiology. But he gave scanty reference to his predecessors.

We know from the listing of titles by such authors as ARISTOTLE, THEOPHRASTUS and DIOGENES LAERTIUS that many treatises on vision, perspective, colors and sense perception had been composed in the classical period of Greece. But in his own treatise on vision, Galen rarely quoted other authors, although prior to his medical studies he had undergone an extensive training in mathematics, philosophy and logic. It was evidently the custom of the times to omit references. Copyrights or priorities had not yet been invented. Thus, we know that the philosopher EPICURUS, the founder of the atomistic school of thought and author of about three hundred scrolls dealing with scientific topics, did not provide a single quotation from other writers [12].

The purpose of the following chapters is to analyze Galen's doctrine of vision according to his studies of the anatomy of the eye, his physiological doctrine of the pneuma, and his knowledge of perspective and optics. Since the results of these three approaches were still imperfect, interesting discrepancies arose.

B. PSYCHOLOGICAL FACTOR IN GALEN'S VISUAL DOCTRINE

The scientists of antiquity could not imagine an action at distance. Therefore, two alternative physiological theories of vision arose: one postulated that an image was traveling from the object of vision to the eye; the other stated that the cerebral pneuma [13] descended first to the eye, then extended forward from the eye to the object, but also carried the image back into the eye, thus causing the visual sensation. Evidently, the Greeks did not separate physics from sense perception and physiology. Physics in the modern sense, encompassing electricity and optics, was not yet known. RONCHI expressed this idea quite well:

12 DIOGENES LAERTIUS, *X:* No. 26 (1959).

13 In the previous study on Galen (SIEGEL, R. E., *Galen's System of Physiology and Medicine*, 1968), it has been explained why Galen distinguished two kinds of pneuma, the *pneuma zotikon*, the *vital spirit* in the blood, and the *pneuma psychikon* in the nervous system, which was defined as *cerebral pneuma (animal spirit)* in order to avoid a psychological interpretation foreign to Galen.

> 'Formerly, the aim of physics had been to explain how the human mind came to know the outside world. Now, the purpose of the new physics is to know the structure and laws of the external world, independently of the observer.'[14]

Already the Aristotelian doctrine of matter and qualities, based on psychological concepts, was poorly supported by empirical, i.e. inductive evidence. In the eyes of the modern observer the ancient doctrine of the four elements and their assumed behavior appears hardly as 'physics', since the senses seemed to indicate only quality-changes in the four basic elements: the perception of temperature was thought to depend upon the qualities of hot and cold; sensation of light and color on the action of the fiery element; taste on changes in the liquid element of water. A certain 'quality' in the sense organ seemed always to respond to a related quality of the object[15].

The failure to distinguish between the physical and psychological events was not an error of logic but the result of a fundamental biological concept. From the vantage point of modern experimental psychology and epistemology, we must realize that many scientists of antiquity included mental awareness in the act of visual perception since they postulated the presence of cerebral pneuma *(spiritus animalis)* in the brain and eye. Even mental processes were projected into the eye which, due to the local activity of the pneuma, was not entirely a 'passive' organ of perception merely transmitting the visual impression to the brain, to which Galen attributed all mental activities in distinction to earlier scientists and philosophers.

The assumed presence of cerebral pneuma in the eye and its extension into space during the act of vision was still interpreted as a psychological act by scientists of the Middle Ages who were indirectly influenced by Galen, since they drew their basic knowledge from EUCLID, PTOLEMY, ALHAZEN and other Arabic scientists. Thus, R. GROSSETESTE's (1168–1253) doctrine of vision postulated that 'the active psychological process of seeing went forth from the eye while material light entered it'[16]. He evidently incorporated the pneumatic optical emission of STOICS, Galen and other scientists of antiquity into

14 RONCHI, p. 15 (1957).
15 DAREMBERG, vol. 1, p. 544; KUEHN, vol. 3, p. 640.
16 CROMBIE, *R. Grosseteste*, p. 114, footnote 1 (1953).

his own doctrine as an explanation for both the material (physiological) and the psychological phase of vision.

The doctrine of vision indeed never became the exclusive domain of a single discipline such as physics, physiology or psychology but remained a complex science involving all three disciplines. The ancient theories of vision remained predominantly psychologic, because the Greeks had failed even to separate the growing science of perspective and refraction from their psychologically oriented doctrines[17]. A strictly physiological approach was as yet impossible, since methods and basic concepts for experimentation on the eye were inconceivable.

C. HISTORICAL SOURCES OF GALEN'S VISUAL DOCTRINE

1. Earlier Sources

Today we distinguish four phases in each act of visual sense perception: the physical phase of the incoming picture; the physiological events during the stimulation of the sense organ; the conduction of the stimulus through specific neural structures to the brain; and the formation of image, representing the psychological reaction of the brain. These four steps in the process of vision must be borne in mind as we study the early attempts to understand visual perception. Prior to Galen, many philosophers, including ARISTOTLE, had not even agreed upon the brain as the seat of psychological and mental function, but they projected conscious sense perception into parts of the body other than the brain. Since most treatises of the early philosophers are lost, we know only very little of their doctrines.

ALCMAEON (beginning of the 5th century B.C.) and HIPPOCRATES (460–355 B.C.) had already localized all mental and emotional functions into the brain. But they made scarcely any assumptions about the physical events of optical transmission through space nor about the processes taking place in eye and optic nerve.

EMPEDOCLES (about 450 B.C.), who was the first Greek philosopher to consider matter as composed of tiny particles[18], explained vision as

17 RONCHI, chap. 1 and 2 (1957).
18 FREEMAN, p. 182 (1953).

a two-way process: as a stream of tiny fiery corpuscles passing first from the eye to the object of vision, like from a lantern, then returning to the eye[19]. ARISTOTLE soon criticized this idea as erroneous[20]. (For details see p. 27ff.)

Although the early members of the atomistic school were contemporary with the other presocratic philosophers, their basic tenets hardly changed until Galen's time, if we disregard the writings of LUCRETIUS whom Galen never quoted (p. 22). An understanding of the visual concepts of the atomists is important for our analysis of Galen's doctrine of visual perception, not only because we know more about their ideas in this field than of the other Presocratics, but because their concept of visual perception seems not to be as contrary to Galen's as one would assume in view of his usual attitude to the teachings of the atomists. Galen did not adhere strictly to one philosophical school but followed mainly the ideas of PLATO, ARISTOTLE and the Stoics. We will see, however, that the ideas of the atomistic school about the problems of vision were more compatible with Aristotelian views than their other concepts.

2. *The Atomists: A Non-Corpuscular Doctrine of Vision*

Although we read in most treatises on ancient science and philosophy that the founders of the atomistic school, LEUCIPPUS and DEMOCRITUS (about 30 years after EMPEDOCLES), based their visual doctrine on the corpuscular concept, it appears to me more likely that they did not relate optical transmission to a stream of atoms. This opinion is contrary to the customary interpretation of their doctrine. It was, however, already expressed, according to the following quotation, by ALEXANDER OF APHRODISIAS. He referred to a visual emanation without speaking of atoms when he summarized the teachings of the early atomists. This author, a commentator on ARISTOTLE, was also a contemporary of Galen:

'Images of some kind and of appearance similar to the object leave

19 FREEMAN, p. 197; DIELS-KRANZ, 31 B 84 and 89.
20 ARISTOTLE, *De sensu*, 437 b 23 and 438 a 3.

the object of vision in continuous stream and arrive in the eye, thus causing visual perception.'[21]

DEMOCRITUS seemed to have assumed that some kind of emanation from the object causes an imprint[21] on the medium in space[22]. Only this 'image' *(eidolon)* was perceived by the eye, he thought, since the original object could not be apprehended directly, as was the case with the other senses. DEMOCRITUS made the statement that this traveling image 'changed the air', the medium between the object of vision and eye, by presenting itself as three-dimensional[22] *(stereos)*. This statement conveys the idea that the visual impression did not depend on the transmission of minute particles but on an alteration of the space between eye and object. The term 'air' did not imply air as an element but, in a figurative manner of speech, indicated here 'space', since he considered the cosmos as a vacuum. Thus, DEMOCRITUS' doctrine of vision appears obviously not to imply the transfer of atoms from the object to the eye (see p. 21, 22).

It was already evident to this early Greek philosopher that an optical image *(eidolon* or *deikelon)* must necessarily have coherence in order to preserve its shape. The preservation of a definite arrangement during optical transmission could not be explained by the random motion of atoms which the atomists otherwise postulated. There is also

21 SIEGEL, *Theories of vision*, p. 146 (1959); DIELS-KRANZ, 67 A 29.—DEMOCRITUS declared that we see an image *(eidolon)* of the object due to an impression *(emphasis)* on the air, which only is a stamped pattern *(typousthai)* due to an unspecified 'emanation' *(aporrhoe)* issuing from all objects (DIELS-KRANZ 68 A 135; also KIRK-RAVEN, p. 421, No. 587).—THEOPHRASTUS (350 B.C.; *De sensu* No. 50) did never mention that DEMOCRITUS spoke of atoms emanating from objects toward the eye. The same applies to ALEXANDER OF APHRODISIAS (ca. 200 A.D.), *De sensu* No. 56, 12, in reference to LEUCIPPUS and DEMOCRITUS (KIRK-RAVEN, p. 422, No. 588). See also FREEMAN, p. 311 (1953). See also p. 19 and footnote 29.

22 DEMOCRITUS' idea that the image in the air becomes three-dimensional *(stereon)* and spatially contracted *(systellomenon)* became later a basic tenet of the Stoic doctrine of pneumatic transmission (KIRK-RAVEN, p. 421, No. 587; DIELS-KRANZ 68 A 135, No. 50). The Greek term *stereos* has been translated by me as 'three-dimensional' and not, as by most other authors, as 'hard'. PLATO used it in the sense of three-dimensional (*Theaetetus*, 148, and *Republic*, 528 a, b). This translation is supported by the *Greek–English Lexicon* of LIDDELL-SCOTT and the *Classical Greek Dictionary* (Follett Publ. Co. Chicago 1927). Further discussion see p. 19, footnote 29. DEMOCRITUS spoke also of *deikelon*, representation (DIELS-KRANZ, DEMOCRITUS, B123). *Systellomenon* refers to the decreasing size of the image on its way to the eye (perspectively; see p. 102).

no evidence that the later atomists attributed vision to a stream of atoms escaping, without internal order, from the object of vision.

We find the non-corpuscular concept of visual transmission also in the writings of the post-Aristotelian philosopher EPICURUS. (ARISTOTLE, died, aged 63, in 321 B.C.) Our knowledge of EPICURUS (342–270 B.C.), the next principal representative of the atomistic school, depends mainly upon the writings of DIOGENES LAERTIUS[23]. From my own studies and interpretation of this writer, it does not follow that EPICURUS stated directly or unambiguously that vision was mediated by a stream of atoms flowing from the object of vision to the eye. But he did write that '*something*' *(ti)* originated from the surface of the object and travelled toward the eye[24]. EPICURUS, however, did not indicate clearly what he understood by this expression. An amended translation of this passage of the text of DIOGENES LAERTIUS (see below) suggests that EPICURUS' doctrine of vision was not altogether different from that of the non-atomistic philosophers, although the opposite is nowadays commonly believed. This revised interpretation can also be supported by referring to Galen who did not indicate that EPICURUS wrote of a corporeal image[24].

Like other writers of antiquity, EPICURUS only said that the illuminated object induced a definite three-dimensional *(stereos)* pattern in the space between object and eye. Naturally, the picture *(eidolon)* had to maintain its original form while passing through space. EPICURUS employed the word *stereos* or *steremnios* to indicate a three-dimensional character of the transmission. It is strange that this term has been commonly translated as 'hard', although PLATO[22] had already employed

23 The modern analysis of the ancient atomistic doctrine relies predominantly on the writing of LUCRETIUS, who lived in Rome during the first century B.C. Although Galen mentioned EPICURUS quite frequently in his books, we cannot find any reference to LUCRETIUS in the index to Galen's work, nor did I encounter his name in Galen's treatises. Interpretation of LUCRETIUS' poem shall therefore be omitted in this study of Galen's doctrine of sense perception (see also p. 22).

24 We have no reason to deduce a corpuscular doctrine from THEOPHRASTUS' statement about visual emanation and formation of a picture in space (*aporrhoea*, and *typousthai*). This agrees with Galen's statement, see also p. 21; footnotes 21 and 27, referring to KUEHN, vol. 5, p. 643.—The KUEHN edition omitted two words which we find in the manuscripts: It should read: *ho d'Epikouros apephenato agein. Kai poly ge toutou kreitton ho Aristoteles, ouk eidolon somatikon alla poioteta di'alloioseos . .* The words *apephenato agein* are missing in the KUEHN edition (vol. 5, p. 643, line 3). I want to thank Prof. PH. DELACY of the University of Pennsylvania for his advice on this question.

it to define spatial extension and cubic numbers. In its modern counterpart, *stereoscopy* means the visualization of a three-dimensional extension in space but not the density or hardness. The Greek term for hard was *skleros* which we still use in medical terms such as *arteriosclerosis*.

The following is the revised translation of EPICURUS' letter to HERODOTUS:

> 'A continuous stream *(rheusis)* comes off the surface of bodies. However, no diminution is observed because of refilling. This flow maintains the position and arrangement of the atoms in the three-dimensional body for a long time, although occasionally it is thrown into confusion. And sometimes patterns *(systasis)* [this does not indicate "films"] are formed very rapidly in the surrounding [space; not "air"] because they do not require replenishment in depth; and there are other modes *(tropoi)* by which such appearances *(physis)* may be formed . . . We must also consider that we see and recognize by the entrance into the eye of something from the outside *(epeisiontos tinos apo exothen)*. Because external objects would not impress [on us] their own natural color and form through the air between us and the objects, nor by rays *(aktines)* nor by currents (fluxes, *rheumaton*) issuing from us to the objects as well as by [the entrance of] certain forms *(typos)* [which should not be translated as "film"] entering from the objects into our organism, [representative] of similar color and shape and also of a size rendered suitable for entry into the visual organ and the mind [the former hinting at the perspectivic diminution of the picture approaching in an optical cone]. Since this proceeds with a rapid motion, it explains in turn the uniform and continuous impression of the emitting objects and the fact that these impressions retain the relationship of the object proportionally to the impact of atoms from the depth of the three-dimensional object *(ek tes kata bathos en to steremnio)*. And whatever impression we gain by apprehension of our mind or our sense organs in regard to the form *(morphes)* or other properties of the object, the form is particular to the three-dimensional *(steremnion)* [arrangement] according to the [perspectivic] contraction [*pyknoma* from *pyknos*, dense] or the traces of the picture *(eidolon)*.'[25]

25 DIOGENES LAERTIUS, pp. 576, 578, 580; X, 48, 49, 50. See also p. 18, footnote 22 *(systellomenon)*.

We notice how carefully the writer avoided referring to a corpuscular or atomic emanation as medium of optical transmission, but that he tried to explain the concept of a perspectivic contraction of the picture, while approaching the eye, with the maintenance of the internal relation of the picture itself. There is no allusion to LUCRETIUS' idea that the approaching picture is hammered together by the atoms of the air during its transmission.

EPICURUS mentioned that the 'picture' is propagated at an infinite speed, since it did not seem to encounter any resistance. This statement would render the idea of a corpuscular stream still more unlikely. Traveling atoms could hardly be propagated at infinite speed, since the corpuscles of the atmosphere (air) would not allow their unobstructed flow, an objection already raised in antiquity.

Unfortunately, the term used by EPICURUS for the outflow *(rheusis)* of the image has often been erroneously translated as 'particles' [26]. This translation, however, would rule out a non-atomistic interpretation of EPICURUS' doctrine of vision. As indicated above, Galen seemed to regard the Epicurean doctrine of vision as an effect only of undefined changes in the optical medium when he wrote:

> 'EPICURUS, however, declared that something passed to the eye. More convincingly ARISTOTLE discussed that not a material *(somatikon)* replica but a qualitative change by alteration *(alloiosis)* of the surrounding air moves from the object of vision to the eye.' [27]

To Galen the concept of 'changes' (*alloiosis;* see also p. 73) evidently seemed not to contradict the basic idea of EPICURUS who spoke of the 'stamping' *(typosis)* of the visual picture onto the air [28]. As a seal

26 BAILEY, p. 408, footnote 1 (1928); see also the translation of DIOGENES LAERTIUS by HICKS, *X:* chapter 48.

27 KUEHN, vol. 5, p. 643; see footnote No. 24 for a corrected reading of the Greek text.—This opinion is further supported by BAILEY, who pointed out that EPICURUS and his followers did not deal with the problem of how a 'film' can disengage itself from a three dimensional object. In fact, BAILEY thought that EPICURUS considered even the concept of an impression as too complicated. He believed that EPICURUS supported the concept of an image *(eidolon)* entering the eye (see footnote 24), but he did not analyze this problem any further.

28 DIOGENES LAERTIUS, *X:* No. 49 (*enaposphragistheito,* to impress); also DIOGENES LAERTIUS, *X:* No. 46. See also footnote 24; similar in sound perception: p. 134, footnote 12.

molded the soft wax, thus an approaching image was believed to transfer its spatial relationship to the medium. The Greek word *typos*[29] meant only pattern or type but did not indicate the transfer of a material on which the original pattern is imprinted. The nowadays often used translation of the term as 'film' implies the contrary idea of a 'skin' composed of atomic corpuscles traveling from the object of vision to the eye of the observer. DIOGENES LAERTIUS wrote:

> 'Again, there are patterns (*typoi*, impressions) which are of the same shape as the three-dimensional bodies of any objects which we see, but of exceeding subtlety *(leptotes)*. For it is not impossible that there could be found in the surrounding [space; the noun is missing in the Greek text; however, the translation as "air" would imply another meaning to the text] some combinations of this kind, adapted for expressing spatial extension and evanescence, or that there are some effluxes preserving the same relative position and motion which they had in the solid bodies. These patterns *(typoi)* [not "films" as translated] we call *eidola* (images) [which were supposed to be three-dimensional, see p. 18]. But since in the vacuum their motions encountered no resistance by countermotions [of atoms], they travel through the whole length in an imperceptibly short time.'[29]

LUCRETIUS (94–55 B.C.) unfortunately spoke of such a membranaceous skin advancing through space. Most modern interpretations of the early Greek atomists are derived from his ideas, although LUCRETIUS' interpretation contradicts evidently the exact wording of the earlier atomists, as was explained above.

LUCRETIUS wrote that either atomic corpuscles *(corpora)* or an undefined matter *(res quaeque)* emanated from the visual objects. He suggested that vision was transmitted in the same manner as sound and odor: 'Corpuscles strike the eye and cause visual perception'[30] *(corpora*

29 DIOGENES LAERTIUS, *X:* No. 46; Loeb. ed., pp. 574, 576 (the translation of HICKS has been modified when indicated).—For the meaning of *stereos* as three-dimensional; see p. 18, footnote 22. In a later paper I will explain that ROGER BACON and other medieval philosophers and scientists accepted the Epicurean doctrine of vision as a non-corpuscular doctrine, i.e. in the same sense as Galen's interpretation (see p. 21). However, modern writers who predominantly consider the Epicurean concept as atomistic hardly refer to the opinion of these medieval writers.
30 LUCRETIUS, IV, verse 217ff.

quae feriant oculos visumque lacessant). LUCRETIUS evidently adapted his wording to the rhythm of his verses, whereas EPICURUS wrote in prose. Since LUCRETIUS seemed compelled to sacrifice clarity to rhythm, we find a certain ambiguity in his terms[31]. LUCRETIUS also failed to differentiate the mechanism of vision from that of other senses, in contrast to EPICURUS and the earlier Greek philosophers. Since Galen did not refer to the writings of LUCRETIUS, these can be disregarded in our analysis of Galen's doctrine.

The idea of a coherent visual transmission without a corpuscular emanation became equally the basis of the doctrine of vision of ARISTOTLE, then of the Stoics, and eventually of Galen. A too rigid classification of the teachings of the Greek philosophers could detract us from recognizing both the subtlety and continuity of their thought about the problem of visual perception.

When EPICURUS and his school assumed that the soul, composed of very subtle atoms, was diffusely distributed throughout the whole body, even the eye[32], they had failed to separate the physiological phase of sense perception from the psychological process of the formation of an image by the mind. EPICURUS not only thought that the unaltered pattern of a recognizable image *(eidolon)* was maintained during the transmission of the optical impression to the eye, but also that it was recognized instantaneously by the soul present in the eye. 'The pictures arise simultaneously *(hama)* with the thought[33].' This statement again indicated not only his inability to differentiate the successive phases of visual perception, a characteristic of Greek 'physiology' (p. 14), but also his failure to appreciate the role of the brain for sense perception and thought.

3. Plato's Visual Doctrine

PLATO (428–347 B.C.) made a similar mistake as the previous philosophers by not separating clearly the physiological and psychological

31 LUCRETIUS, IV, verse 225: *omnibus ab rebus res quae quae* ('something') *fluenter fertur*; in Greek it was *tinos* 'something' (ref. 24).

32 BAILEY, p. 396ff.

33 RONCHI supports this point of view: 'Ces images se forment en même temps que naît la pensée' (p. 24, 1957). The translation of HICKS that the 'production of the pictures is as quick as thought' (DIOGENES LAERTIUS, Loeb ed., vol. 2, p. 577) is incorrect.

aspects of the process of vision. Since he considered the light and the soul to be of identical nature, he postulated a movement of the soul beyond the confines of the eye into space through which the optical image had to travel. His writings were of great importance to the Stoics and to Galen, and, at least, formed the basis of a detailed discussion by these philosophers.

Galen devoted several treatises to the analysis of PLATO's writings, quoting passages from THEAETETUS and TIMAEUS in his 7th book of the *Commentaries on the dogmas of Hippocrates and Plato*. This important treatise will soon be available in English translation thanks to the efforts of Prof. PH. DELACY of Philadelphia [34].

PLATO showed little interest in the exact anatomical description of the eye nor did he present a coherent doctrine of vision, but he dealt only with those aspects which would support his own philosophical ideas. This resulted in an unscientific combination of observation with metaphysical assumption. BEARE, in a thorough study of ancient sense perception, confirmed this impression when he stated that PLATO's physical ideas were submerged in metaphysics [35] and that the nature of light was of less interest to PLATO from the viewpoint of physics and psychology than from that of metaphysics [36]. The following quotation from the TIMAEUS will illustrate PLATO's rather unscientific style:

> 'The spherical form of the head, being the most divine part ... within us, ... should not go rolling upon the earth ... It would be at a loss how to climb over the heights and hollows ... For this reason the body acquired length ... and shot forth four limbs ... They set the face in front ... and constructed light-bearing eyes, and caused pure fire to flow through the eyes ...' [37]

Fundamentally in agreement with the atomistic interpretation of vision, PLATO considered matter as composed of geometrically shaped particles. He stated that the pure fire, resembling the mild light of the day which issued forward from the eye to the object, was composed of

34 I want to thank Prof. PH. DELACY for the great courtesy of letting me read through his manuscript of this translation.

35 BEARE, p. 43 ff. (1906).

36 BEARE, p. 47 (1906).

37 PLATO, *Timaeus*, 44 D–45 B.

corpuscles *(moria)* of a specific shape like those of fire[38]. He wrote that when the light of the sun had aroused the activity of the eye[39] it produced a centrifugal 'stream'[40] of vision to the object seen. This stream meets particles flying from object to eye:

> 'Whenever the stream of vision is surrounded by midday light, it flows out like unto like, and coalescing therewith it forms one kindred substance along the [straight] paths of the eye's vision.'[41]

He believed that vision was maintained principally by an emanation to the eye:

> 'When the kindred fire vanishes into night, the [returning] sensation is cut off.'[42]

In opposition to the earlier philosophers, PLATO stated further that 'vision' depends as much on the outside light as on the activity of the sense organ (i.e. on the emanation from the eye). PLATO's doctrine of vision reflected, however, his compelling interest in the mystical source of biological forces. He wrote:

> 'The power which the eye possesses is a sort of effluence which is dispensed from the sun.'[43]

Thus, according to PLATO, the visual emanation of the eye had its origin in the sun; but during the act of vision it traveled from the eye to the object, and was reflected back to the eye. From there it reached the soul, which he located in the blood and liver, both organs of perception[44]. This doctrine indicated actually a three-fold path of the light: from the sun to the eye, then to the object and back to the eye. It was a rather roundabout way to demonstrate that:

38 PLATO, *Timaeus*, 67 C, D.
39 PLATO, *Republic*, 508 b; JOWETT, vol. 2, p. 370.
40 PLATO may have been influenced by the statement of EMPEDOCLES that the eye is like a lantern, sending forth light by which we see; *Timaeus*, 45 C; also FREEMAN, p. 197.
41 PLATO, *Timaeus*, 45 C, 67 D.
42 PLATO, *Timaeus*, 45 D.
43 PLATO, *Republic*, 508 b; JOWETT, vol. 2, p. 372.
44 PLATO, *Timaeus*, 71 B, 72 C; BEARE, p. 272.

'The sun appears as the author of all visibility in all visible things.'[43]

PLATO hardly referred to other scientific writings of his time, although we know that prior to PLATO many philosophers had written on vision and light[45]. Likewise PLATO did not discuss whether visual perception was localized in the pupil or in other parts of the body[46]. He even failed to recognize the brain as an instrument of the thought and sense impression[47], since he regarded the liver as the principal seat of sense perception[48].

Since PLATO considered color as different from light, defining it as emanation from the surface of objects, he devoted more attention to the theory of color mixtures than to the discussion of the physical nature of light.

In conclusion: PLATO's doctrine did not contribute much to our understanding of Galen's ideas about visual perception, since Galen was interested in the physiological reaction of the various parts of the eye to light, regardless of whether the light was white or colored[49]. Galen followed, however, PLATO's erroneous idea of an emanation issuing from the eye. In other respects, he was greatly influenced by ARISTOTLE, and he disregarded entirely PLATO's assumption of geometrically shaped atoms as carrier of light.

Like PLATO, who did not heed his own advice that the description of nature should be based on the mathematical method[50], ARISTOTLE (384–322 B.C.) failed to apply a mathematical or geometrical interpretation to the problems of vision. Although several other authors had previously written on optical reflection and perspective[51], ARISTOTLE's doctrine of vision represented rather a deductive approach to these problems. It is remarkable, however, that ARISTOTLE was able to outline the basic viewpoints and logical difficulties of an analysis of vision. His ideas still demand our attention and were certainly of considerable importance for Galen.

45 BEARE (1906), gives a detailed analysis of these authors.
46 PLATO, *Timaeus*, 45 D.
47 BEARE, p. 335 (1906).
48 PLATO, *Timaeus*, 71 A, B.
49 White light was called *auge* (brightness).
50 PLATO, *Timaeus*, 47 c.
51 An exception was ARISTOTLE's geometrical analysis of the rainbow as reflection from clouds: ARISTOTLE, *Meteorologica*, 373 a 5–18.

4. Aristotle

ARISTOTLE's concepts on visual perception represented two aspects which he was unable to integrate into a uniform doctrine, since they reflected two logically opposing views: the idea of a transparent medium and the concept of light rays. We later shall see that Galen had similar difficulties in his attempt to formulate his own doctrine of vision.

a) The Transparent Medium

ARISTOTLE refuted the idea of the earlier philosophers that the picture of an object seen in the pupil of a person was an essential phase of the visual process. He wrote:

> 'The image is visible [in the eye] because the eye is smooth [like a mirror]. It exists, however, not in the eye but in the observer; for this phenomenon is only a reflection.' [52]

Furthermore, ARISTOTLE wrote in refutation of PLATO's doctrine that it was unreasonable to propose that we see by something issuing from our eye. ARISTOTLE disagreed also with PLATO's idea that extraneous light was fused in space with light coming from the eye, or that fusion took place in the eyeball. He wrote:

> 'What is the meaning of light coalescing with light?' [53]

ARISTOTLE advanced as his own doctrine of vision that a spacefilling medium of undefined nature underwent certain changes during the act of vision. He called this medium the 'transparent' *(diaphanes)* [54]; he assumed that by the influence of light on this medium the exact features of the visual object were transmitted to the eye. His idea that an internal 'motion' *(kinesis)* of this medium produced vision [55] greatly influenced Galen's visual doctrine.

52 ARISTOTLE, *De sensu*, 438 a 7.
53 ARISTOTLE, *De sensu*, 438 a 29.
54 In Greek an adjective with an article becomes a noun; thus *diaphanes* can represent, according to the context, either an adjective or a noun.
55 ARISTOTLE, *On the soul*, 418 b 1 – 419 a 25; 438 a 14.

ARISTOTLE postulated that the transparent medium itself remained stationary and invisible, even while receiving and transmitting visual images. He believed that vision could only occur when this medium was activated by light of whatever source. ARISTOTLE wrote that most light came from the sun, although there were exceptions such as luminescent bodies.

'Light is the energy, the active force of the transparent.'[56]

He described the concept of the 'transparent' in the following manner:

> 'What we call "transparent" is not a characteristic feature of air, water or of any other substance, but is their common nature and activity; it pertains inseparably to these substances ...'[57] 'A transparent medium exists. As transparent I understand not what is visible as such, to say it simply, but what becomes visible by the color belonging to something else.'[58] 'We see only colors; every color corresponds to motion in the medium which by its own nature is transparent.'[59] 'Light as the activity of this transparent medium results in color.'[60] 'It is wrong to state with EMPEDOCLES that light travels and passes unnoticed at times in the space between earth and its [cosmic] surroundings.'[61]

ARISTOTLE's idea of an undefined medium was only a postulate which he conceived in order to explain optical transmission[62]. His idea was comparable to the now obsolete 19th century concept of ether which likewise postulated a stationary weightless substance, continuous

56 ARISTOTLE, *On the soul*, 418 b 10ff., *(energeia)*. He also defined it as *dynamis*, activity, of the transparent.

57 ARISTOTLE, *De sensu*, 439 a 22ff.

58 ARISTOTLE, *On the soul*, 418 b 3.

59 ARISTOTLE, *On the soul*, 419 a 10. See also chapter on color p. 79, 82.

60 ARISTOTLE, *On the soul*, 418 b 10. The modern ether was considered as matter but not corporeal, which was a logical paradox (abbreviated).

61 ARISTOTLE, *On the soul*, 418 b 21.

in itself and all-permeating, as the substrate of the light rays[62]. Like the Aristotelian 'transparent', this modern ether was thought to be activated by light. The propagation of the change in the ether seemed not to be impeded by transparent bodies, since it passed through them as if passing through empty space.

The Stoic philosophers modified ARISTOTLE's idea, speaking of a change in a pneumatic medium as 'tension' *(tonos)* (p. 39, 89). But in all three hypotheses, ARISTOTLE's transparent medium, the Stoic's pneuma[63] and the modern ether, the transmission of an optical picture did not depend upon the traveling of corpuscles or of another agent.

ARISTOTLE wrote that since the 'transparent' permeated substances such as water or air[64], it also had to be present in the eye because, according to ancient doctrine, the eye contained a large share of water[65]. 'The transparent is the nature and property of all substances'[66], were the words of ARISTOTLE.

SAMBURSKI[67] suggested that the optical medium of the ancient philosophers was the prototype of the electromagnetic field. This comparison, however, is not justified, since ARISTOTLE had neither the intention nor the methods of applying a mathematical interpretation which is the principal feature of modern science.

Galen's concept of transmission of the optical impression through space had one aspect in common with ARISTOTLE's idea about the 'transparent': he did not postulate a material transport of the image but only a 'change' *(alloiosis)* of the medium as an essential condition for the propagation of light. Galen's idea was, however, derived from the concept of the *cerebral pneuma* issuing from the eye (p. 72), but not from ARISTOTLE's assumption of a transparent medium.

62 ARISTOTLE assumed that 'light' traveled instantaneously through space ('infinitely fast'). He ruled out that corpuscular transmission could be equally instantaneous, a reasoning quite correct for his primitive method of observation.
63 See p. 37 ff.
64 ARISTOTLE, *On the soul*, 418 b 8.
65 ARISTOTLE, *De sensu*, 438 a 14; 425 a 1.
66 ARISTOTLE, *De sensu*, 439 a 21: *(Koine physis kai dynamis tois allois somasin enhyparchei.)*
67 SAMBURSKI (1959), p. 37.

b) The Principal Organ of Perception

Since ARISTOTLE did not yet recognize the brain as the seat of mental perception [68], he was greatly mistaken about the localization of the psychological functions connected with visual perception. Galen understood the role of the brain as the seat of perception and criticized ARISTOTLE and PRAXAGORAS for considering the heart as the origin of the nerves and as the seat of the soul. ARISTOTLE was, however, inconsistent in expressing his opinion as to whether visual impressions were conducted to the brain or to the heart. In some passages he denied anatomical connections between eye and brain [69], in others he admitted that eye and brain were contiguous (especially in reptiles) [70]:

> 'The eyes are indeed, like the other sense organs, set upon passages *(poroi)* . . . The purest part of the liquid around the brain is secreted through those passages which are . . . leading from the eyes to the membrane around the brain.' [71]

He apparently never understood fully the connection between the brain and the sense organs, since he even thought that the acoustic nerve terminated under the skull in a hollow space. But ARISTOTLE, at least, understood that the visual image was propagated from the eye into the optic nerve, although he had failed to find the central termination of the optic nerve.

ARISTOTLE explained nerve conduction as the propagation of a qualitative change along the nerve, like heat traveling through a suitable conductor. We read in ARISTOTLE's *On sleep and waking* that the other sense perceptions are also mediated by qualitative changes in the nerves [72], an idea later taken up by Galen. We have to recognize that

68 KUEHN, vol. 5, pp. 200–203. Since ARISTOTLE noticed that touching the brain did not provoke pain reaction in the experimental animal or in a wounded person, he concluded that the brain could not be the seat of pain perception, or for that reason of any form of perception. Further, only parts of the body containing blood seemed to be able to perceive. Therefore, the heart appeared to him the foremost organ of sense perception. (ARISTOTLE, *Progression of animals*, 656 b 16ff.; 656 a 29; 666 a 12; 647 b 25; see also CLARKE, 1963.)

69 ARISTOTLE, *Progression of animals*, 652 b 2.

70 ARISTOTLE, *History of animals*, 503 b 13.

71 ARISTOTLE, *Generation of animals*, 744 a 1–12.

72 ARISTOTLE, *De somnis et vigilia*, 457 b 1.

one of the fundamental differences between ARISTOTLE's and Galen's sense physiology was based on Galen's correct understanding of the role of the brain for all mental processes. Although 500 years had elapsed since ARISTOTLE, Galen was still compelled to devote much time and energy to refuting the time-worn argument that the seat of conscious sensation was in the blood, in the sense-organs or even in the heart. Galen had clearly established that the nerves terminate in the brain but not in the surrounding membranes or blood vessels [73], yet this fact remained widely unrecognized by his contemporaries. Galen had also to struggle against ARISTOTLE's idea that conscious perception can take place in a peripheral organ such as the eye [74].

c) Light Rays

ARISTOTLE did not raise the question of how the transparent, space-filling medium the *diaphanes*, carried separate linear light rays if it had to be considered as a material agent, continuous in all directions and undivided. However, ARISTOTLE could not avoid discussing optical rays as separate linear entities in contrast to the indivisible *diaphanes*, when he referred to binocular vision. ARISTOTLE understood that the optical image was transmitted to the eyes in such a manner that every point of the object was projected to an identical point of each eye. Based on this concept, ARISTOTLE explained double vision in an almost modern sense, stating that it arose when the incoming rays did not terminate at corresponding points of both eyes. This idea presupposed a rectilinear propagation of light rays, since it was evident that distinct points in the eye could only be connected with the object of vision by linear rays. We read in the *Problemata* (probably composed by ARISTOTLE's successor at the Peripatetic school):

73 See p. 6ff.
74 ARISTOTLE (*De sensu*, 438 b 11; also *Historia animalium* 491 b 20) stated that the 'dark' is surrounded by white, which denotes the sclera. The 'dark' was therefore the iris. But it could not mean the darkness of the pupil as it has been suggested, since he wrote: 'The central part of the eye includes the moist part whereby vision is effected; it is termed the pupil, and the part surrounding it is called the "dark" *(melas)* [i.e. the iris].'—'There must be, therefore, [in the eye] a translucent medium and as this is not air, it must be water. The soul or its perceptive part is not situated at the external surface of the eye; but the eye is the sensory instrument of the soul, which is obviously somewhere within.' (*De sensu*, 438 b 8ff.)

'Why do images appear double if the eyes stand apart [as in squinting]? Is it because the movement [of the transparent medium] does not arrive at the same point of each eye? Therefore, the soul thinks that it is seeing two objects when it sees double.'[75] '[The positions of] those eyes who receive the optical impression on the same spot [in each eye] are not distorted. They are mostly fixed in their position.'[76]

Aristotle was, of course, not referring to corresponding points of the retina but to points on or in the lens or the vitreous. The consideration of points implied that light rays were the transmitting agent, since only rays could terminate in points. Aristotle had also observed that 'when a man presses a finger under the eye, a single object will appear double'. Galen quoted this experiment, but did not express as clearly as Aristotle that visual perception required the coordination of identical points of both eyes toward the object.

In his description of the rainbow, Aristotle also referred to distinct light rays, being aware that the rainbow was caused by sunlight reflected from innumerable droplets of the clouds:

'The reflection is from the mist that forms around the sun or the moon . . . Since reflection takes place in the same way from every point, the result is necessarily a circle or a segment of a circle; for if the lines start from the same point and end at the same point and are equal, the points where they form an angle will always be a circle.'[77]

Could Aristotle assume that reflections from points are anything else but rays?

Galen ran into the same difficulty as Aristotle, when he tried to combine the doctrine of a homogenous optical medium with the rules of optics, which are based on the assumption of linear rays. But we will see that he admitted the existence of rays, whereas Aristotle avoided this issue almost entirely.

75 Aristotle, *Problemata*, 958 b 11.
76 Aristotle, *Problemata*, 958 a 13. We know that normal eyes are mostly in the position of a physiological angle of convergence. They are only in parallel position when facing distant objects.
77 Aristotle, *Meteorologica*, 373 a 2ff.

ARISTOTLE must have further observed that light was propagated in a straight course from object to observer, since looking through a tube seemed to prevent scattering of the light rays and to intensify the perception. It did not occur to ARISTOTLE that, by elimination of extraneous light, people could see the stars more clearly from the bottom of a deep well[78]. He wrote:

'Distant objects would be seen best if there were something straight and continuous extending from the eye to the object of vision, such as a tube. Motion [i.e. of the *diaphanes*] issuing from the object would not be scattered.'[79]

He was apparently influenced by the analogous observation that the ear canal offers protection against the scatter of the motion of air. But these observations did not necessarily prove the existence of light rays.

Before we proceed to a discussion of Galen's doctrine of vision, we must also become acquainted with the research in optics and perspective after ARISTOTLE. Several references to EUCLID prove that Galen was familiar with EUCLID's treatises.

5. Euclid's Geometrical Laws Applied to Optics

EUCLID (323–285 B.C.), who lived in Alexandria, was born one year before the death of ARISTOTLE (in 322 B.C.). We are told by PROCLUS, a Neoplatonic philosopher of the 5th century A.D., that the treatise *Optics*[80] attributed to EUCLID is most likely authentic. Apparently, the genuineness of literary sources was already in question. This treatise proves that many laws of perspective and a doctrine of vision based on linear light rays had been established 400 years before Galen.

EUCLID postulated that not only the sun but also artificial sources of light emit linear rays. Experimenting with a small source of light and two separated boards placed at the same level he found, when he perforated the first board at the height of the center of the lamp, that

78 ARISTOTLE, *Generation of animals*, 780 b 22.
79 ARISTOTLE, *Generation of animals*, 781 a 9ff.
80 EUCLIDE, *L'optique et la catoptrique* (ed. of 1959) (catoptrics deal with reflection from mirrors).

the light could pass through the perforation of the second board only when the light source and the two openings were in one straight line[81].

In the first definition of his *Catoptric*[82] EUCLID described that visual rays issuing from the eye were directed only toward the object of vision where they terminated, but that they did not spread diffusely (as presumably light does in a transparent medium). EUCLID wrote:

> 'Let us suppose the visual rays as straight lines terminating at the [two] ends [i.e. one end at the eye and the other at the object seen].'[83]

But EUCLID stated that the rays issuing from one point in the eye diverge toward the object, each ray remaining separate. Thus, space could not be filled by the rays as it would be by the Stoic pneuma. The sum total of all rays leaving the eye formed a cone. The base of this cone represented what a modern physician would define as the visual field. EUCLID did not specify where in the eye the end-point of the cone was located, but he considered that, at least, part of the base of the cone coincided with the surface of the object of vision.

EUCLID thought that a small but remote object may escape attention since it occupied the space between two light rays. Therefore, we could not perceive simultaneously all the letters on a page, or we might fail to see a needle lying on the floor unless we directed our view straight at this object[84]. When EUCLID thought that small objects were often not noticed, he mistakenly substituted a physical for a psychological explanation.

According to EUCLID's doctrine, visual perception was a discontinuous process, since it relied on the assumption of distinctly separated diverging light rays. He wrote:

> 'No length seen is seen at one time in its entirety . . . But the visual rays are displaced so fast that it appears to be seen at once.'[85]

81 VER EECKE, *Recension de l'optique par Theon*, p. 53 ff.

82 Probably edited by THEON in the 4th century A.D. (SARTON, vol. 1, p. 367, 1953); see also VER EECKE, p. XXIX.

83 VER EECKE, p. 99.

84 THEON's introduction to EUCLID's *Catoptric*, VER EECKE, pp. 53–56.

85 EUCLID's *Catoptrique* (VER EECKE), pp. 57–58 (I. Proposition). EUCLID did not search for a photosensitive area of the eyeball.

EUCLID's concept implied that the central visual rays of the cone[86] had to move with the eye swiftly along the surface of the object in order to explore all of its parts. The object appeared uniform to an observer only because of the high speed of movement of the eye. EUCLID tried to overcome by this assumption his failure to understand that perception also required the lateral rays.

EUCLID's treatise indicated the eye itself as the point from which all visual rays emerge. In his text he always indicated the position of the eye by a letter, like the points in geometrical diagrams. EUCLID left no clue as to whether he thought that the visual rays came from a point in the pupil, from the lens or from a point behind the lens. To EUCLID as mathematician the eye was merely a crossing point of visual lines. When speaking of light rays, Galen adopted the same method, regarding the eye as a geometrical point (p. 94).

Preoccupied with the concept of divergent rays of the visual cone, EUCLID failed to point out that parallel rays leading away from the eye appear to meet at a point which we define today as the vanishing point. He suggested this rule in his 6th proposition:

> 'Parallel lines when seen from a distance appear to be an unequal distance apart.'[87]

Although he recognized that the distance between parallel lines appeared to become smaller with increased distance from the observer, EUCLID might have been hesitant to speak of a 'vanishing point'. It would have been exactly the opposite to the 'point' in the eye from which the visual rays supposedly issued toward the object of the vision. Evidently, the concept of EUCLID's diverging visual rays reversed the rule of modern perspective according to which parallel lines converge at a point opposite to our eyes.

EUCLID's failure to grasp that perception is only possible when the rays travel from the object to the eye merely illustrates his disregard of the physiological aspects of vision. He followed the tendency criticized by KEPLER (p. 11) that mathematicians were entirely disinterested in the anatomy and function of the eye, whereas natural scientists

86 The ancients, and especially Galen, believed that the central ray of the visual cone was most essential for perception; see p. 87–92.
87 COHEN and DRABKIN, p. 259; VER EECKE, p. 2.

tended to neglect mathematics. KEPLER deplored this attitude even of his own contemporaries.

For centuries after EUCLID, the understanding of the problems of vision hardly advanced[88]. Although our knowledge remained fragmentary because of the enormous loss of ancient documents, the few references in the surviving literature point at a lack of important research in optics prior to Galen.

During the Hellenistic period, geometrical optics became an applied science, helpful for instance in manufacturing various types of mirrors, even the huge reflecting mirrors designed for producing fire at the focal point. In this manner, ARCHIMEDES of Syracuse put the attacking Athenian fleet to rout by conflagration (212 B.C.). Only one important work on optics has been preserved, as a monument of Greek science of this period, PTOLEMY's *Optics*, which was written shortly before or during Galen's time.

6. Ptolemy's Optics

This famous astronomer lived in Alexandria during the 2nd quarter of the 2nd century A.D. simultaneously with Galen. Unfortunately, the important first chapter of PTOLEMY's *Optics* which dealt with the theory of vision has been lost. The other parts of this treatise explain, in great detail, the laws of perspective and of monocular and binocular vision. Like EUCLID, he stated correctly that the optical cone of each eye is directed to the object of vision at an angle equal to that of the other eye[89]. He recognized that the 'symmetry' (i.e. the symmetrical position) of both cones guarantees the perception of a single picture during binocular vision. While doing research on double vision, PTOLEMY observed that the second image could more easily be suppressed during lateral than vertical displacement of one eye. Without referring to PTOLEMY, Galen undertook similar experiments (p. 106ff.).

In contrast to EUCLID, PTOLEMY did not believe that the transmission of an image by light rays would cause an interrupted picture, because a remote object did not appear 'full of holes'. But like ARISTOTLE and EUCLID, PTOLEMY thought that only a central visual ray issuing

88 We know from the writing of DIOGENES LAERTIUS that numerous treatises on optics written prior to EUCLID have also been lost.

89 He called it the optical pyramid instead of cone; see footnote 251.

from the eye arrived at a point of the object opposite to the observer before it returned along the same path to the eye[90]. From other positions, however, the returning ray appeared subject to the laws of refraction[91]. Although PTOLEMY had established, in many experiments, the almost correct angle of refraction of rays passing from one medium into another[92], he did not correctly apply this knowledge to the interpretation of the passage of light through the different media of the eye, especially the lens.

The incomplete Latin translation of PTOLEMY's *Optics* (ed. by LEJEUNE) is the only text which has survived. Thus we are forced to reconstruct PTOLEMY's views on vision from the scattered remarks in those chapters of this work which were devoted mainly to the analysis of the laws of refraction and perspective. Although Galen did not quote from PTOLEMY's treatise as he did from older medical texts, there was a definite chance that PTOLEMY's treatises were of great influence on Galen or, at least, that Galen discussed many ideas and observations which he found in PTOLEMY's treatise. It also appears possible that both scientists based many conceptions on a common source unknown to us.

Very little is known about the treatises on vision by other physicians of the classical and Hellenistic period, men of such importance as PRAXAGORAS, HEROPHILUS[93] or ERASISTRATUS, whose influence in other fields Galen repeatedly admitted.

When in his earlier years and prior to his medical education Galen had studied philosophy under tutors hired by his far-sighted father, he was greatly influenced by the Stoic teachers. An understanding of the Stoic views on sense perception therefore appears indispensable.

7. *Pneumatic Concept of the Stoics*

The Stoics explained vision by emanation of a continuous pneuma, unlike PLATO's stream of fiery corpuscles. They conceived that this weightless agent penetrated the entire nervous system (*pneuma psychikon, cerebral*

90 PTOLEMY, *Optics*, p. 88, III, 3.

91 PTOLEMY's *Optics*, p. 184.

92 LLOYD, p. 56.

93 HEROPHILUS only described the optic nerves which he believed to contain a central canal *(poros)*; both optic canals seemed to join at the chiasma for exchange of pneuma. KUEHN, vol. 3, p. 813; KUEHN, vol. 5, p. 206.

pneuma; in Latin *spiritus animalis,* from *anima,* the soul). During the act of vision, this pneuma was thought to issue first from the eye through space to the object, where it underwent changes in its structure *(alloiosis)* which were conducted back to the eye and brain. This doctrine did not stipulate the emanation of material corpuscles, but the propagation of a 'tension', of an alteration in space comparable to the propagation of the image through ARISTOTLE's transparent medium. The 'transparent' of the Aristotelian school was supposedly present in eye and space prior to the act of sense perception. The Stoic pneuma, however, had first to flow from the eye into the space between eye and object. Common to both doctrines was the concept that visual transmission did not require the transfer of matter. Evidently, the Stoic doctrine did not advance the science of optics and perspective nor did it make use of the extant anatomical knowledge which had been acquired since ARISTOTLE's time.

It is difficult to speak about a consistent or uniform doctrine of sense perception of the Stoic philosophers, since their teaching had already begun at the time of ZENO (third century B.C.) and was still flourishing at Galen's time. The Stoic who exerted the greatest influence on Galen was CHRYSIPPUS. He was born in Cilicia (Asia Minor) in 280 B.C. and died 207 B.C. CHRYSIPPUS, like the later Stoic philosophers, believed that vision consisted of the two phases which have been discussed above. He wrote that a pneumatic stream proceeding from the object *(aistheton)* strikes upon the sense organ *(aistheterion)*. He called this impact 'sensation' in a narrower sense *(aisthesis)*. At the same time, the mind as the ruling part of the soul sends out the spirit *(pneuma)* to meet the impact of this pneuma. This combined operation was also termed 'sensation'[94].

This doctrine was not merely a modification of PLATO's theory of vision which postulated that these phenomena were based on a corpuscular emanation. According to our limited sources, CHRYSIPPUS spoke of changes in the medium between the object and eye by a subtle alteration of its structure *(alloiosis)*[94] during the process of vision. This is important, since Galen frequently used the same expression as CHRYSIPPUS *(alloiosis)* for this hypothetical change in the transparent medium during the act of vision[95].

94 ARNOLD, pp. 130–131.
95 For the Stoic visual doctrine: see also CHERNISS (1933).

Aetius (5th century or beginning of the 6th century A.D.) confirmed that, according to Chrysippus, vision took place by an emanation of pneuma which, after striking the air, changed its own state of tension; further, that the pneuma initially went forth from the pupil in the form of a cone toward the object of vision, fusing with the optical rays issuing from the object. The emanation of the eye was thought to be of a fiery nature. Aetius understood, however, that this was not a physical fire, although it was thought to be related to the fourth element, the heat of fire[96].

Independently, however, of metaphysical speculation, the pneumatic philosophers believed that the change of the space-occupying pneuma *(alloiosis)* into a state of higher tension could explain the physical nature of visual transmission. They compared this effect on space to the motion of a 'stick', since the area of increased density *(tonos)* seemed to assume the form of a straight and narrow tube. This comparison suggested that optical impressions were physically transmitted. Aristotle had explained all sense perception as contact or 'touch': 'touch' *(haphe)* as the basic perception of the hand; taste as the 'touch' of food on the tongue; sound as the 'touch' of air to the membranes; finally, the idea of an optical 'stick' reduced vision to the 'touch' of a circumscript column of 'space' upon the sensory parts of the eye (see also p. 31 ff.). Thus, vision appeared also as a mechanically transmitted event.

It seems to us that the simile of the stick had probably two other sources: a stick was used by the blind to recognize by touch otherwise unrecognizable objects; secondly, the Stoics may have used the simile of the stick metaphorically: the diameter of a stick, reduced to an infinite thinness, could be compared to an optical ray[97]. The Stoic scientists may also have considered the narrow bundle of central rays in the visual cone as a 'stick'. Some Stoics spoke indeed of linear propagation of light, although they still maintained the doctrine that 'light' is a change in structure of the homogenous transparent medium. They regarded, therefore, the pneuma and the light rays as the essence of vision[98]. There is an indication in the ancient literature that the Stoics considered the theorem of infinite thinness in order to find a compromise between the concepts of pneuma and light rays (see p. 88).

96 Von Arnim, vol. 2, p. 233, No. 866; Plato had a similar idea. See also Siegel, Galen's System of Physiology and Medicine, p. 141 ff. (1968).

97 Von Arnim, vol. 2, p. 233, No. 865; also Kuehn, vol. 5, p. 642.

98 Arnold, p. 249, footnote 68.

Galen modified the Stoic pneumatic doctrine of nervous activity and visual perception with regard to his advanced anatomical knowledge of the eye. He was also aware that scientific progress depended upon a clear distinction between the optical features of visual perception and the hypothetical events in eye and brain. But like his predecessors, he was unable to reconcile the pneumatic doctrine with the rules derived from optics and perspective.

D. GALEN'S DOCTRINE OF VISION

1. Galen's Description of the Eye (Figure 1)

It has been stated by other medical historians that Galen's doctrine of vision was that of PLATO partly influenced by ARISTOTLE and the Stoics[99]. This view greatly underestimates Galen's contributions to the problems of vision. In the preceding chapter a detailed history of the important theories of vision before Galen was given, because Galen attempted to integrate the traditional concepts with the results of his own observations, his modification of the pneumatic doctrine and with the rules of geometry, optics and perspective.

99 CHERNISS, p. 161.

Figure 1. Schematic view of the human eye.

The *optical* [*visual*] *axis* (interrupted line) extends from the middle of the *cornea* through the center of the *lens* to the *macula* which is known today as the most light-sensitive spot of the retina. The entrance of the *optic nerve* into the eyeball, slightly medially from the macula, is called *optic disc*. Because of an error in dissection Galen believed that the central ray (axis) entered the optic nerve directly at the disc. The *retina* covers the inside of the eye from the optic disc and terminates in a circle to which the lens is attached by delicate fibrous connections and where also the membraneous *iris* and *uvea* are attached.—Galen assumed that pneuma, entering the retina from the *central canal* (Fig. 5) of the optic nerve, traveled via the fibers of the retina and through its attachments to the uvea and lens, rendering the latter light-sensitive.—The idea of a direct path of light rays to the optic nerve was the basic concept of Galen's geometrical analysis of vision, whereas the observation of connections between retina and lens formed the basis of Galen's pneumatic doctrine of vision.

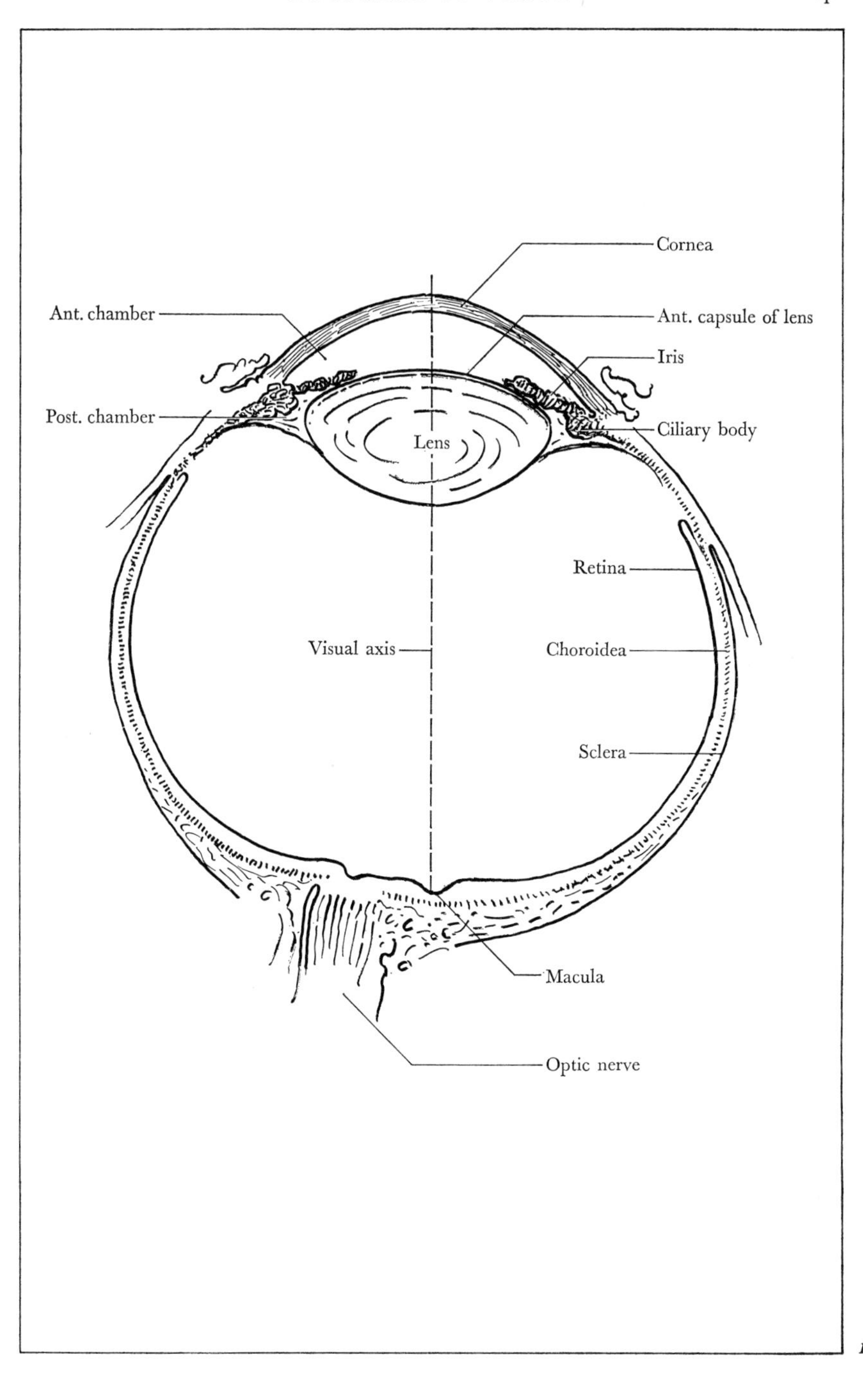
Cornea
Ant. chamber
Ant. capsule of lens
Iris
Post. chamber
Ciliary body
Lens
Retina
Visual axis
Choroidea
Sclera
Macula
Optic nerve

The long series of anatomical studies of earlier physicians [100] which can not be discussed here, culminated in Galen's description of the structure of the eye. His account appears quite correct, if we consider that he dissected only the eye of animals. Furthermore, none of the earlier physicians had formulated a comprehensive doctrine of vision, at least no such text has been preserved. We find one treatise which Galen wrote on the structure and function of the eye in the Greek edition of Galen's works [101]. A second predominantly anatomical treatise, which has been discovered only in recent times, was preserved in the Arabic translation [102]. Both treatises are now available in English translation [101].

We shall better understand Galen's doctrine of vision when we first discuss his anatomical description of the eye which was mainly derived from studies on the ox (Fig. 1).

Galen marvelled at the anatomical structures of the eye which, he thought, was an instrument of such perfection that it only could have been invented by a superior mind. He spoke in teleological terms of the creator (*demiourgos*, literally craftsman). But it would be wrong to consider Galen's teleology as vitalistic and unscientific. Modern anatomists still relate morphological design to function, pointing out without hesitation that most structures are adapted to a certain purpose. To mention only a few instances: the small perforations, visible only under the electron microscope in the basement-membrane of the capillaries evidently represent a filter for the blood serum into the chambers of the eye; likewise the transparency of the media of the eye or the plasticity of the lens do not need further explanation.

Galen's description of the anatomy of the eye was extremely detailed [103]. He recommended the use of special instruments for dissection, advising his readers how to prepare the eye, and even the whole animal, for the study of the eyeball. He stated that death of the animal through suffocation by a noose or by immersing in water

100 For studies of HIPPOCRATES and RUFUS, see SHASTID (1917).
101 SHASTID (1911): Also M. T. MAY (1968). Details, see on page 200.
102 DUCKWORTH, W. L. H., *Galen on anatomical procedures*, book 10 (Cambridge Univ. Press 1962), English translation of the Arabic text. A German translation of the Arabic text has been published by SIMON, M., *Sieben Bücher der Anatomie des Galen* (Hinrich, Leipzig 1906). Vol. 1 is a reproduction of the Arabic text; vol. 2 its German translation. The optical chapter is in vol. 2, pp. 25–60.
103 KUEHN, vol. 3, p. 760ff.; vol. 14, p. 712; DUCKWORTH, pp. 33–50.

produced a better visibility of vascular details by distention of the veins[104].

A passage from Galen's treatise conveys the painstaking research and the meticulous dissection technique which he employed:

> 'An observer, looking at the cornea of a living animal, might perhaps conclude that its composition is identically the same in every detail up to its superficial surface. But the matter is not so. When you examine a horn which one can split into fine layers . . . or alabaster which one sets in windows, you will notice, as each slice is removed, the color of that which lays behind it. So in the eye you will look from the first layer to the color of the layer which lies beneath it . . . You must train yourself so . . . that the incision [of the cornea] should run in a straight line, passing through the center of the cornea . . . Next, draw the two margins of the incision apart with two sharp hooks . . . incise this layer, a sort of covering for the cornea . . . set free a second and then a third layer . . . But as for the remaining stratum of the cornea, it ruptures immediately if you apply the scalpel . . . and there flows out from behind it a liquid . . . that is colorless.'[105]

We know today that the cornea consists of several layers which can be differentiated under the microscope. Behind the cornea but separated by the narrow space of the anterior chamber is the iris. When the fluid of this chamber escapes, the space between cornea and iris becomes obliterated, as Galen wrote:

> 'When the fluid has escaped . . . the cornea is superimposed upon another layer, of which the color is the same as that of the "front view" of the eye [i.e., the iris] before you dissect the eye . . . Its central aperture [the pupil] is circular in many animals like in man, but in some animals it is slit-like as in cattle . . . Within this aperture you can see the ice-like[106] humor of the lens . . . but less hard than ice. You can see that the grape-like layer [the posterior wall of the iris, which we call today *corpus ciliare* or *uvea*; from the

104 DUCKWORTH, p. 38.
105 DUCKWORTH, pp. 34, 35.
106 The lens was compared to a chip of ice floating on water. Therefore it was described as a congealed watery humor.

Latin word *uva*, grape] is attached to and blended with the cornea only at the cornea-scleral junction ... To both again [i.e. iris and sclera] the lens attaches itself.' [107]

Galen described further the anterior and posterior chambers of the eye:

'You will see ... the space between cornea and iris [anterior chamber] ... and also the space between iris and crystalline lens [posterior chamber] ... The iris is free from the crystalline lens and from the cornea ...' [108] (Fig. 1).

Galen next described that the retina as an extension of the optic nerve formed threadlike connections to the lens. He considered the retina as the pathway of visual perception when he wrote:

'As soon as the optic nerves reach the eyes they unfold and expand, surrounding the vitreous humor on all sides like a garment, and finally each optic nerve attaches itself to the crystalline body [of the lens] which is the essential organ of vision ...' [109] 'The [optic] nerve spreads out and becomes shaped like a net.' [110] [The Greek term for the retina is *amphiblestroeides*, since it looks like a fisherman's net; literally: that what is thrown around].—'The humor which is covered by the net-like tunic ... is called vitreous, because the consistency of its structure resembles molten glass and its tint is the same as that of clear glass ... The crystalline lens, however, is an even clearer white [i.e. transparent] in color than the vitreous humor ... it is spherical with the exception that it is slightly flattened transversely (Fig. 1 and 5) [111]. Consequently, many anatomists called it lentiform, wishing thus to compare its form to a lentil-seed ... A delicate sheath envelopes the lens externally ...

107 DUCKWORTH, pp. 35, 36. See figure 1.
108 DUCKWORTH, p. 37. Galen knew that the anterior and posterior chambers communicate through the pupil. He raised the question whether the chambers are filled with air or with a watery fluid. (DAREMBERG, vol. 1, p. 621; Galen, *De usu partium*, X, 5; KUEHN, vol. 3, p. 781.)
109 DUCKWORTH, p. 39; also KUEHN, vol. 3, p. 760ff. (condensed).
110 DUCKWORTH, pp. 39, 42, 43, 188.
111 Slightly changed according to the translation by SIMON, p. 35ff.

It is on this [i.e. the anterior capsule of the lens] that we observe our image, just as when we see it in a mirror, when we look into the eye of a person close to us (see p. 49). That sheath clothing the lens . . . has been found to resemble the distended membrane of a froth-bubble . . . it is thinner than a spider's web.' [112]

When Galen described the vascular choroid membrane, surrounding the retina externally, he made the error of assuming that the retinal blood vessels enter from the choroid [113]. They actually are derived from the central retinal artery and vein which enter through the optic nerve. Their branches do not anastomose with those of the choroid membrane [114].—Further details of Galen's anatomy of the eye have to be omitted. They are accessible in English translations (see p. 42, notes 101 and 102); also Galen's detailed studies of the external structures of the eye, such as the muscles, the eyelids, the lacrimal glands and ducts (which Galen discovered). The latter have no direct relation to the visual problems to which this chapter is devoted.

2. *Galen's Complementary Approach to the Problem of Visual Perception*

Combining the teaching of his predecessors with his own observations and ideas, Galen tried to integrate their different concepts into a logical system. Basic contradictions between the pneumatic and geometrical interpretation of the visual process were already evident in the writings of the earlier Greek scientists and philosophers. Further errors and difficulties resulted from Galen's lack of understanding optical refraction and from his failure to distinguish the physiological from the psychological processes of perception. Principally, however, these difficulties arose from the incompatibility of the two traditional doctrines, the pneumatic concept and the laws of optics and perspective. Therefore, Galen formulated two different approaches to the problems of vision. After a brief survey of the principles of both doctrines, each will be

112 Duckworth, pp. 37–41 (condensed).
113 Kuehn, vol. 3, p. 763.
114 The vortical veins of modern terminology; Polyak, pp. 598, 623, 663; fig. 365 (1957).

submitted to a detailed analysis: first Galen's pneumatic, then his geometrical analysis of vision.

a) The Pneumatic Concept

Galen drew his pneumatic concept of vision mainly from the Stoic philosophers who explained the transmission of the optical impression as the propagation of a structural change in the pneuma occupying the space between the object and the observer. In addition, Galen had accepted PLATO's concept of a two-way action manifest during the act of seeing. Galen said it consisted first of the emission of pneuma from the eye to the object, then of the return of the pneuma carrying the image to the eye. However, Galen rejected PLATO's atomistic interpretation of sense perception. Galen's pneumatic doctrine of vision did therefore not contain any atomistic concepts. This even applies to Galen's interpretation of the visual doctrine of the atomists themselves (p. 46).

As discussed above, Galen was justified to regard EPICURUS' concept of visual transmission as a non-corpuscular doctrine. Therefore, EPICURUS' idea of the transfer of a complete image through space *(eidolon)* appeared not even to contradict Galen's pneumatic principle (p. 19). Likewise, ARISTOTLE's concept of a transparent medium indicated that a correct replica of an object was transmitted to the observer without transfer of matter.

It was important to Galen to sustain a pneumatic doctrine of vision, since only on this basis could he correlate the action of the pneuma during the visual process with his doctrine of nerve conduction. Galen considered that vision was mediated by the same agent which he assumed as carrier of all cerebral activity, the *pneuma psychikon.* (This term has been translated as '*cerebral* pneuma', since both the Latin term *spiritus animalis* and its literal translation into English as *animal spirit* might suggest 'animal' and thus easily lead to a wrong understanding (see also p. 4). The theory of conduction by an active pneuma or by qualities carried by pneuma formed the basis for Galen's idea of optical transmission through space, the eye and the optic nerve, although Galen did not give a clear answer to the question of nerve conduction. His views have to be briefly summarized.

Galen offered three possible mechanisms: nerve conduction could be mediated by the movement of a stationary pneuma in the central canal of the nerves; or by the pneuma emitted from the brain into the nerves during stimulation; or by the transfer of a powerful action *(dynamis)* [115], which he related to the presence of a quality, along the nerves during stimulation. Although Galen declared it impossible to give a definite answer, he regarded the transfer of an immaterial 'power' along the nerves as most likely. For the optic nerve he apparently assumed that the stimulus also propelled pneuma through both the central canal and the substance of the nerve. Galen's pneumatic doctrine aimed at a uniform explanation by assuming that the pneuma was not only the agent of optical perception by the eye but also its physical carrier through the nerves and the space [115].

b) The Geometrical Concept (Figure 1)

Based on anatomical observations, Galen had suggested that the sensory pneuma in the lens of the eye received the first optical impression, and that the stimulus was then conducted from the lens by connecting fibers to the retina and from there to the brain. But Galen was unable to correlate this idea with the rules of perspective and optics. He, therefore, formulated an alternative doctrine of vision based on the concept that light traveled rectilinearly through the eyes via the optic nerves to the brain. Galen explained this doctrine of vision in the treatise *The function of the parts* [101]. He also tried to give experimental evidence to these ideas or, at least, to relate these concepts to the geometrical treatise of EUCLID whom he quoted on several occasions. Some reference to the geometrical approach concerning the problems of vision can also be found in Galen's extensive *Commentaries to the dogmas of Hippocrates and Plato* (see p. 48). Further, it appears quite possible that Galen based many of his ideas and experiments concerning optics and perspective on the treatises of PTOLEMY. The principal concepts of both EUCLID and PTOLEMY have been outlined briefly in a preceding chapter but will be related to Galen's treatise again in the respective parts of this discussion.

115 See p. 71. *Dynamis* and *pneuma* were often used in the same sense; see SIEGEL, *Galen's System of Physiology and Medicine*, pp. 183, 192 (1968).

c) Galen's Writings on Vision

Galen discussed the problems of vision in *De usu partium* (*The function of the parts of the body*, book 10; translated into French by DAREMBERG, vol. 1, pp. 607–651; into English by SHASTID in the *American Encyclopedia of Ophthalmology*, vol. 11, p. 8590–8622 [from the German of KATZ]; KUEHN, vol. 3, pp. 759–841). Galen discussed first the anatomy of the eye and the pneumatic doctrine. The geometrical discussion starts with chapter 12 (KUEHN, vol. 3, p. 812). An English translation of *De usu partium* has been published in 1968 by Mrs M.T. MAY (Cornell Univ. Press). This book appeared after my manuscript was sent to the publisher and therefore could hardly be considered.

Galen's *Commentary on the dogmas of Hippocrates and Plato* has not yet been translated. These commentaries are usually referred to as '*Placita*'. Prof. PH. DELACY, Philadelphia, is working on the translation of these commentaries for the *Corpus Medicorum Graecorum*. In this extensive treatise (KUEHN, vol. 5, pp. 211–805) Galen's geometrical doctrine is mentioned on page 626ff. (book 7, chap. 5).—I want to thank Prof. PH. DELACY for the courtesy of letting me read his manuscript.

A description of the anatomy of the eye can be found in DUCKWORTH, *Galen on anatomical procedures*, pp. 27–50 (Cambridge Univ. Press 1962). The same Arabic text was translated and annotated earlier in German by SIMON, *Sieben Bücher der Anatomie des Galen*, vol. 2 (Hinrich, Leipzig 1906). The first volume is a photoprint of the Arabic text.

It is possible to ascertain the period during which Galen wrote these chapters, since he compiled two autobiographical treatises [116]. We learn from these that both the chapters in '*De usu partium*' [117] and the '*Commentaries*' were composed during a brief period. We can rule out an evolution of Galen's thought on vision over an extended time.

We have to admire Galen's intellectual honesty, since he not only formulated two separate doctrines but even explained the motivation for writing the second doctrine. He stated that, since initially he had neglected speaking of perspective, refraction and the role of optical rays, he felt obliged to write a separate chapter on the geometrical analysis, although he anticipated from past experience a lack of in-

116 Galen, *De libris propriis*, KUEHN, vol. 19, pp. 8–48; *De ordine librorum suorum ad Eugenianum*, KUEHN, vol. 19, pp. 49–61.

117 KUEHN, vol. 3, pp. 758–841. (*De usu partium*, book 10.)

terest in geometrical and mathematical explanations[118]. He complained that most people present at his lectures preferred the principles of the pneumatic doctrine of visual perception.

3. Pneumatic Doctrine of Vision

a) Pupillary Image

An observation which greatly puzzled the philosophers of antiquity was the appearance of an image of outside objects in the eye of another person. Most ancient doctrines of vision presented a faulty explanation of this pupillary image. The early Greek philosophers had never made it clear whether this image was formed on the cornea or deeper inside the eye (i.e. on the surface of the lens). Usually they thought that vision was located in the pupil[119]. Galen's opinion about this problem was different from that of his predecessors which we will discuss first.

To an observer, the image visible in the eye of another person is upright and seems to fill the entire pupil. The Greek word for pupil is *kore* (literally 'girl'). It appears possible that this term was derived from the Greek word *korennymi*, to fill out, indicating that a picture fills the opening in the iris, the pupil. But the Latin translation of the Greek word *kore* also indicated 'little girl', since the Romans used the term *pupilla* or *pupula*, the diminutive of *pupa*, 'girl'. The word *pupilla* had also the meaning of 'puppet' which suggests an image, the replica of a person.

ARISTOTLE interpreted the image in the pupil as the result of reflection not by the lens but by the water in chambers of the eye when he wrote:

> 'The image is visible [in the eye] because the eye is smooth; it exists, however, not in the eye but in the observer; for this phenomenon is only a reflection.'[120]

118 KUEHN, vol. 3, p. 812.
119 ARISTOTLE, *On the soul*, 413 a 2; BEARE, p. 80.
120 ARISTOTLE, *De sensu*, 438 a 7. *Although* BEARE, p. 80, wrote that *kore* is the crystalline lens, the Greek text and a quotation from THEOPHRASTUS justify us to say that they regarded *kore* as the pupil; see also p. 45.

ARISTOTLE thought that the optical impression of this image was carried by the watery humor from the pupil to the optic nerve and from there into the blood, the seat of perception:

> 'The visual organ proper is composed of water, yet vision appertains to it not because it is so composed but because it is translucent, a property common to both water and air. Water is more easily confined and more easily condensed than air; therefore, it is that the pupil, i.e. the eye proper consists of water.' [121]

ARISTOTLE based his still primitive idea of visual reception by water of the eye on the observation of a watery flow from an injured eye from which either the fluid of the chambers or, in more serious injuries, the vitreous can escape (see Fig. 1). ARISTOTLE, however, did not think that the pupil itself was black because it was filled with a colorless watery fluid. He may have been familiar with the passage in HIPPOCRATES' treatise 'On the flesh':

> 'The so-called pupil of the eye only appears black, because it is situated in the depths of the eye and surrounded by dark membranes ... It is not black on inspection but colorless and transparent.' [122]

Thus ARISTOTLE believed that the active process of vision was located in the pupil since its water appeared light receptive.

Contrary to ARISTOTLE, Galen did not consider that the pupil took an active part in the process of vision, since it represented only a hole in the iris, filled with a clear fluid. But like ARISTOTLE, Galen was convinced that the 'little picture' which appears in the eye of another person was reflected. He thought, however, that this reflection took place at the anterior surface of the lens. We know that a mirror-image can become visible on the frontal aspect of the lens after the cornea has been experimentally removed. But we have no indication that Galen performed this experiment on animals. He only said that the anterior lenticular capsule seemed to act both as a mirror and sensory organ, according to its particular structure, since Galen wrote:

121 ROSS, 438 a 13ff.
122 LITTRÉ, vol. 8, p. 607.

'The anteriorly protruding part of the lens which touches the *uvea*[123] *(rhagoeides)* is enclosed by a shining and delicate membrane. The pupillary image is contained on it as on a mirror. But it is thinner and more glistening, exceeding [the brightness of] any mirror.'[124]

It should be mentioned that the Romans used not only plain metal mirrors but also glass mirrors in which the rays were reflected by a metal plating behind the glass. It is suggested that the name *crystalloeides*, glass-like, applied not only to the substance of the lens but also to the transparent and colorless capsule separating the lens from the fluid contents of the eye. Galen compared the lenticular capsule indeed to the glass lining of a mirror. He continued in the same chapter:

'The capsule attached to the lens is smooth, shining and glistening. The [structure] next to it is vascular, soft, black and perforated [the iris and the ciliary body]: vascular in order to supply the cornea freely with nourishment; soft in order to be attached to the lens without injuring it; dark in order to gather the light together and lead it toward the pupil; perforated [by the pupil] that the brain can send [the cerebral pneuma] outward.'[125]

It seemed to Galen that the dark pigment of iris and choroid held the light together to prevent scattering of the rays passing through the pupil to the glistening anterior capsule of the lens[126].

b) Lens and Visual Image; Ciliary Body

Galen thought that the curved surface of the lens was perfectly adapted to its alleged function of visual perception, since it presented a larger anterior surface to the incoming optical image than either a flat

123 The *uvea* is the posterior surface of the iris; it also is called ciliary body.
124 KUEHN, vol. 3, p. 787; also ref. 112; and HIRSCHBERG (1919).
125 KUEHN, vol. 3, pp. 787–788; SHASTID, p. 8602; *De usu partium*, book 10, chap. 6.
126 *De usu partium*, book 10, chap. 3; DAREMBERG, vol. 1, p. 619; KUEHN, vol. 3, p. 769ff. In KUEHN, vol. 7, p. 92, Galen mentioned that even the inner blue lining of the sclera is light-repelling. I could observe it on the eye of the ox, beneath the retina and choroid membrane, covering the sclera with the blue color of mother-of-pearl.

or a perfectly globular lens would do (Fig. 1). He had found the width of the lens larger than its thickness (i.e. its depth from the anterior to the posterior capsule). Since Galen also observed that the anterior capsule of the lens was heavier than its posterior covering[127], he deduced that the image on another person's eye was formed on the anterior capsule of the lens. We know, however, that this image is actually formed on the surface of the cornea.

Galen attributed no real significance for the perceptive act to the image visible on the lens of another person. Likewise, ARISTOTLE had considered that this replica of the object of vision was not perceived before it had arrived via the bloodstream in the center of mental awareness, the heart[128]. Incidentally, ARISTOTLE did not discuss how the picture could be transmitted from the eye into the heart, since, according to ancient doctrine, the blood was supposed to flow in both veins and arteries toward the periphery of the body, exactly opposite to the alleged course of the sense impression in the blood vessels.

The observation of an image reflected from the anterior surface of the lens suggested to Galen that the lens had the specific task of receiving and transmitting the visual impression to the brain. But Galen gave no indication how to explain that the shape and color of the object were preserved in this tiny image during the transmission through pneuma in space, nor did he suggest how the identity of its form was preserved while the 'image' traveled from the lens to the perceiving brain and its ventricles. Anatomical considerations seemed, however, to support his concept that the first stage of visual perception was located in the lens.

Galen based his doctrine about the sensitization of the lens by pneuma on a detailed anatomical study of the eye of the ox. I reviewed Galen's observation by examining ox-eyes fresh from the slaughterhouse. The Galenic instructions for the dissection of the eye of the ox proved a valuable guide[129]. On careful preparation it was possible to extract the entire vitreous intact, the lens on its center. The ciliary body, marked by its radial black spokes, was still attached to the periphery of the capsule of the lens. The flat ciliary body is a disk-like vascular structure which occupies in the intact eye the space between the sclera and the posterior part of the iris, covering the outer circumference of the iris from behind. The ciliary body is attached with its

127 These membranes are almost microscopically thin.

128 BEARE, p. 80; ARISTOTLE, *On sleep and waking*, 456 a 7.

129 DUCKWORTH, pp. 30–43.

outer margin to the retina, whereas its inner margin faces the lens, to which it is connected by innumerable fibers. During preparation of the specimen the connections between ciliary body and lens remained intact (as stated above), but those to the retina were torn, since the retina remained inside the eyeball covering the choroid membrane. The fibers of the retina could easily be distinguished from their origin in the optic nerve, to their very end where they fuse into the ciliary body [130] (see Fig. 2).

The radially arranged black spokes of the ciliary body form a very beautiful pattern and seemed to Galen as a convincing demonstration of the functional connections between retina and lens. It was Galen's mistake to infer a functional relation from these anatomical relations. These structures are easily visible on the ox-eye, since it is larger than the human eye.

Modern books on the anatomy of the human eye describe other delicate fibers extending from the retina to the capsule of the lens along the ciliary body as meridianal fibers of the corpus ciliare. These originate likewise at the retina and terminate at the capsule of the lens. They were first described by ZINN in 1755 as *zonula fibrosa* and bear his name since that time. It is unlikely that Galen could have seen these extremely delicate terminal extensions of the ciliary body which suspend the lens.

In summary, Galen believed that the outside picture was received by the lens as the principal receptive part of the eye. The lens exhibited two features which could not be explained in any other way: firstly, it was connected to the retina by the black fibers of the ciliary body, and secondly it was believed to be sensitized by pneuma descending from the brain through these same attachments. These structures were thought to maintain the flow of pneuma in two directions: from the brain through the optic nerve and retina to the lens and backwards from the lens to the brain over the same channels. Thus, Galen stipulated the retina as a purely conductive instrument. This concept of the

130 Galen defined the corpus ciliare with its fibers as *rhagoeides*, from the Greek word *rhax*, grape; the Latin term *uvea* is still used in modern anatomy to indicate the bulging posterior protrusions behind the iris. We must assume that Galen considered the iris (in the modern sense) and the ciliary body *(uvea)* as a functional unit in regard to the pupillary movements (miosis and mydriasis, i.e. the narrowing and opening of the pupil, see p. 67).

retina carrying the optic impression to the brain was a major discovery, although it outlined only one part of its true function, since the retina contains also the light-sensitive cells from which conductive fibers lead to the optic nerve. These, of course, were unknown to Galen. The sensory function of the retina was not discovered for another 1400 years.

By postulating that the optical impression traveled from the retina through the optic nerve to the brain, Galen not only refuted ARISTOTLE's assumption that the sense perceptions were carried into the heart, but for the first time, he stressed the importance of the retina for visual perception. However, he failed to explain how the optic stimulus was conducted in a sufficiently orderly fashion from the eye to the brain to form a mental picture. Only a most delicate analysis by modern microscopical technique could demonstrate that the optical fibers terminate in the occipital area of the brain, where the points of the retina are represented on the cerebral cortex in a manner corresponding to their topographical arrangement in the eye.

It has been mentioned (p. 45) that Galen believed in the possibility of an alternative pathway by which the visual impression is led in a straight line from the cornea directly to the optic nerve. This concept could hardly be compatible with Galen's pneumatic doctrine of vision, because it implied a rectilinear conduction of optical rays through the lens, the vitreous and the optic nerve. This second doctrine also made it superfluous to assume the lens as the seat of percep-

---

Figure 2[1]. Lens and uvea seen from the rear: Attachment of lens to retina.

Galen believed that the radially arranged pigmented streaks of the *uvea*, between *retina* and *lens*, served as channels for the *cerebral pneuma (spiritus animalis)*. This pneuma was supposed to enter the retina from the central canal of the *optic nerve* (see Fig. 1), then travel through the retinal fibers and the radial attachments of the *uvea* (black lines in this photograph) into the *lens* which was thus thought to become photosensitive. If one removes the *vitreous* from the ox eye intact, the lens lying on its center, the uvea exhibits the beautiful black lines which are arranged radially. The *iris* lies below the uvea and is not visible in this picture.

1. Sclera—2. Choroid membrane—3. Uvea (ciliary body)—4. Indicates the radial spokes—5, 6. Lens.—AVERROES (12th cent.) restated this Galenic doctrine (EASTWOOD).

[1] This figure is a reproduction from a photograph in SISSON and GROSSMAN (1953) with the permission of the publishing house (Saunders, Philadelphia).

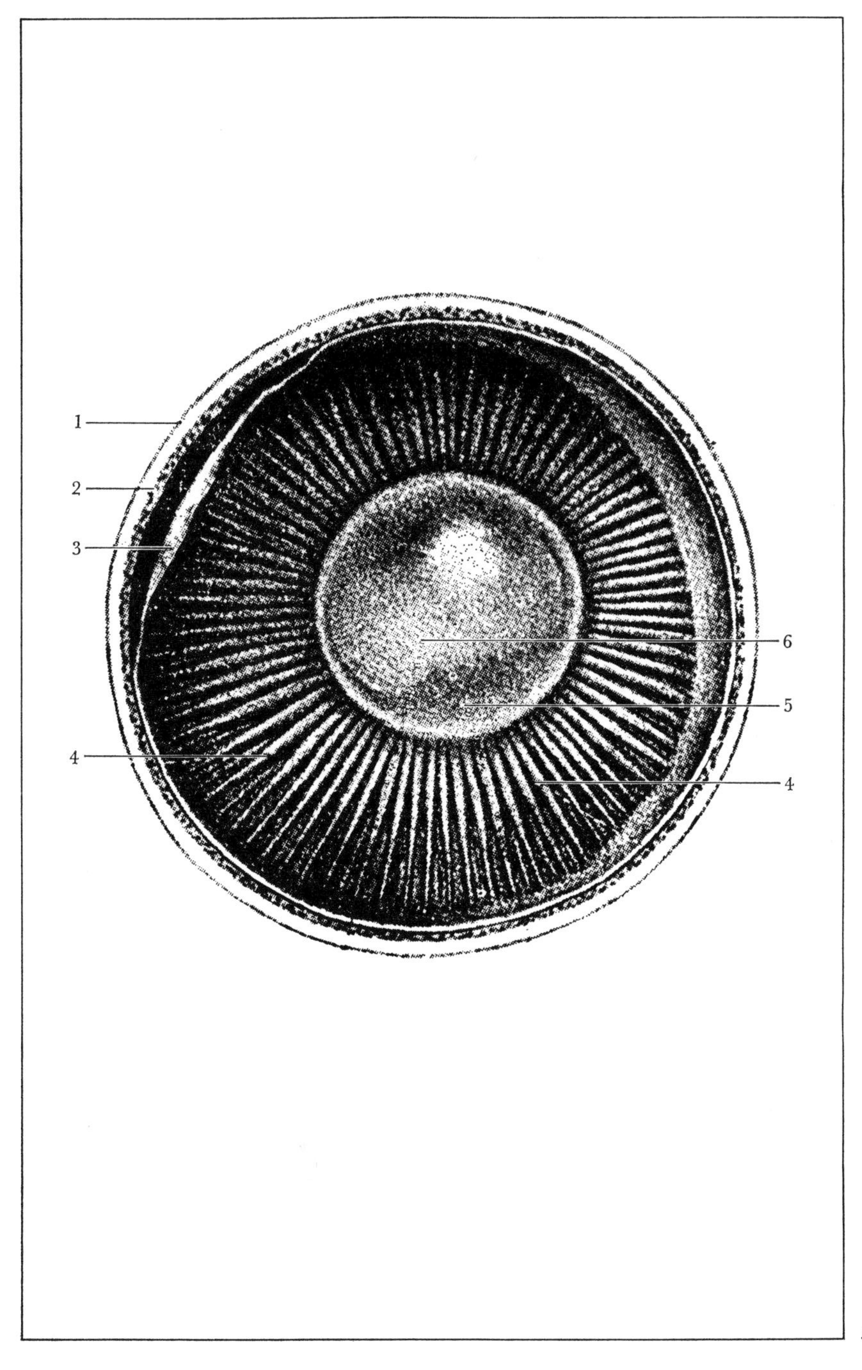
1
2
3
4
6
5
4

tion. It further discarded the idea that the visual impression was conducted via the ciliary body to the retina as the pneumatic doctrine postulated. But before we proceed to an analysis of these ideas, other aspects of the pneumatic doctrine have to be discussed.

c) The Retina

Galen correctly described that the retina is the innermost layer of the eye surrounding the vitreous, and that it is covered toward the outer layer of the eye by the choroid membrane. The latter, in turn, is protected by the sclera. Although he did not examine the development of these membranes during fetal life, as he had done on heart and blood vessels, Galen considered all coats composing the wall of the eyeball as extensions of the meningeal membranes and of the brain. Thus he described the sclera, the external white protective layer of the eye, as the derivative of the dura mater; the vascular layer inside the sclera, the choroid membrane, as the derivative of the vascular arachnoid membrane; finally he correctly understood the retina, the sensory part of the eyeball, as a derivative of the optic nerve and, therefore, of the brain itself. He wrote:

> 'In appearance the retina is indeed like a net, but not like a membrane at all, neither in color nor in substance. One would surely believe, if one everywhere detached it and rolled it together, that one had before oneself a detached portion of the brain. Its chief function, that for which it was sent down by the brain, is to perceive the alterations which occur in the crystalline body [lens] and to communicate these [to the brain]. In addition, of course, it has to conduct and deliver nourishment to the vitreous humor. For this reason, the retina contains a very large number of arteries and veins, many more and of greater size than would be appropriate to its own mass; for with all the nerves which originate in the brain, there passes down a portion of the chorion-like meninges provided with arteries and veins.'[131]

131 SHASTID, pp. 8591–8592 (modified); KUEHN, vol. 3, p. 762. We have to assume that Galen described here the vascular connections of the ox eye.

It is of interest that a modern textbook of anatomy describes the retina in terms similar to those by which Galen indicated it as part of the brain:

> 'That part of the retina which contains the optic fibers is called the cerebral layer of the eye.'[132]

On dissection of the eye of the ox, one can see that the retina is a mesh of thin fibers which, with the help of a fine probe, can easily be lifted up from the bluish colored sclera. On careful inspection, one can indeed recognize, exactly as Galen stated, that the fibers of the retina converge toward the optic nerve. Also its color was, as Galen described, that of the brain. The name which Galen gave to the retina was chosen to indicate 'a net thrown about' the vitreous *(amphiblestroeides)*.

We know today that the lens, as a purely optical instrument without nervous connections, only focuses the incoming rays on the particularly sensitive area of the retina, the macula. According to Galen, however, the lens was not an agent of refraction but the principal organ of visual perception because of its content of cerebral pneuma.

Galen assumed that the pneumatic optical impression was first received by the lens, then conducted through the attachments, mainly through the ciliary body, via the retina and optic nerve to the central nervous system. (We cannot suppose that Galen was able to visualize the almost microscopical retinal attachments to the lens which are called zonula ZINNII and were discovered in the 18th century.) The relation between the retina, the ciliary body and the lens are reproduced in Figures 1 and 2.

Galen never considered an optical point-to-point projection of the image on the retina. The idea of a *camera obscura* was still completely unknown. Because of his failure to understand the optical behavior of the lens he had paid such great attention to the image visible on the surface of the eye (which he thought was reflected by the anterior capsule of the lens, p. 52–54).

Prior to reception of the visual image by the optic system the cerebral pneuma had to be conducted to the eye in order to sensitize its structures for the reception of the optical image. The central canal of

132 BROESICKE, pp. 703, 708 (1912). The retina is called in German Netzhaut (Netz means net). The retina of some animals contains even ganglioncells.

the optic nerve, opening toward the vitreous, suggested the passage of some cerebral pneuma into this clear substance and even to the lens by further diffusion. Most of the pneuma seemed, however, to follow the nerve fibers of the optic nerve which, after entering the eyeball, spread around the vitreous as retina, terminating at the outer circumference of the lens, which 'looks like a flattened sphere'. The vitreous had only an important role in Galen's geometric doctrine of vision, when all light rays had to pass through the center of the eye. The geometrical analysis of the visual process will be explained in the second part of this chapter (p. 86ff.)[133].

In the frame of Galen's pneumatic visual doctrine, the retina represented the only important link for the conduction of the optical impression to the brain. In fact, the optical image already reached the brain matter on entering the retinal fibers which structurally appeared to Galen as an extension of the brain itself like all the other nerves (both cranial and peripheral). Galen wrote:

> 'The lens *(crystalloeides hygron)* is the primary organ of vision. It is one of the constituents of the eye and is composed of uniform parts. It is altered *(alloiosthenai)* by something pertaining to the colors of the outside object which the animal perceives.'[134] 'Dividing itself and flattening out its neural substance the retina surrounds the vitreous and grows into the lens as its maximum circumference.'[135]

Thus, the lens appeared as the principal organ of vision to which the retina was subordinated.

> 'The lens is the organ of vision, and all the parts of the eye are created for its sake.'[136]
>
> 'The optic nerves ... flattening out [as retina] surround the *hyaloeides hygron (vitreous)* and go into the lens *(emphyomenoi eis to*

133 KUEHN, vol. 5, pp. 623–625 *(Placita)*.—In the second part of this chapter, it will be explained why Galen did not consider only the retina as link in transmission of an optical image. The visual process was analyzed as the passage of rectilinear light rays through cornea, lens and vitreous to the optic nerve. It was unknown that rays were refracted by the lens. This doctrine disregarded the role of the pneuma.

134 KUEHN, vol. 10, p. 48.

135 KUEHN, vol. 5, p. 624.

136 KUEHN, vol. 10, p. 118.

> *krystalloeides)* . . . which is the principal organ of vision . . . colorless, brilliant and clear.'[137]

To the modern observer, however, the retina appears more important than the lens, because an operatively removed lens can be replaced by eye glasses. Since the ancients were not familiar with lenses, an injury or even the loss of transparency of the lens appeared as equally as deleterious to vision as a lesion of the optical nerve; diseases of the retina were unknown.

Galen wrote that both the vitreous body and the lens are colorless, since they were without blood vessels. We know today that this was correct, because the blood vessels are carried by the surrounding structures (choroid membrane, iris, uvea). Galen erred, however, when he attributed only to retinal vessels the function of supplying nutrition to lens and vitreous by diffusion (*diadosis*, transfer) and of secreting the fluid in the anterior and posterior chambers of the eye.

d) Optic Nerves and Chiasma
(Figures 3 and 4)

Long before Galen it was known that the visual stimulus passed through the eye into the optic nerve. As mentioned before, Galen had postulated two alternative pathways of the image to the optic nerve: one by pneuma via the lens and the retinal fibers, the other by light rays directly and rectilinearly through the lens and the vitreous. The latter pathway will be discussed in the chapter on optics and perspective. At present, we will confine ourselves to the role reserved for the optic nerves in the pneumatic doctrine of vision.

After some vague references to earlier studies, mainly by HEROPHILUS (4th century B.C.), Galen described correctly that both optic nerves, on their course to the brain, are crossed at the *chiasma* (from the Greek letter *chi*, written X). He explained that the chiasma, as we still call it today, was almost at the center of the base of the skull, directly in front of the pituitary gland (hypophysis), since this was 'the only space adapted for it'. The main reason for the crossing of the

137 DAREMBERG, vol. 1, pp. 607–608; KUEHN, vol. 3, pp. 760–761; *De usu partium*, book 10, chap. 10, 1.

two optic nerves was the assumed exchange of the pneuma travelling along their central canal. Galen believed that in this manner the separate pictures coming from each eye could be fused into a single impression. After the chiasma, the picture was supposedly carried forward by the pneuma through the further course of the optic nerve (we call the extension of the optic nerve between the chiasma and the brain the optic tract). Galen thought that this nerve (i.e. the optic tract) entered finally the lower part of the lateral ventricle of each side[138].

He stressed the difficulties of a correct dissection of the structures at the base of the brain:

> 'If one did not prepare this specimen carefully, one might easily believe that the [optic nerves] really cross *(epallattesthai)* each other and run one above the other. That, however, is not the true state of affairs. But as soon as they have touched each other inside the skull they unite their central canals; they then separate immediate-

138 KUEHN, vol. 5, p. 613; vol. 3, pp. 813ff. and 835ff.; DAREMBERG, vol. 1, p. 648. The Greek text (KUEHN, vol. 5, p. 613) indicates that an opening *(trema)* into the cerebral ventricle was practically invisible, even in oxen. For ALCMAEON, see DIELS-KRANZ 24 A 8; also SIEGEL (1959); DAREMBERG, vol. 1, p. 648. Probing with hog bristle: DUCKWORTH, p. 186 (1962).

Figure 3. Anatomy of the visual and olfactory system according to Galen (human brain, ventral aspect; schematic drawing).

Galen wrote that the *optic nerve* continues after the crossing at the *chiasma.* This part of the nerve is called *optic tract,* a modern term not used by Galen. It terminates at the *thalamus* (i.e. chamber) of the *lateral ventricle.* Galen considered the thalamus as part of the lateral ventricle (as its Greek name already suggests), whereas we understand the *thalamus* as a large agglomerate of ganglion cells on each side of the brain medially from the lateral ventricle. Galen said that the optic nerves entered the *thalamus* of the lateral ventricles, because the ventricles were the seat of conscious perception.—The olfactory system of the brain consists of the *olfactory bulb* which is small in man, large in animals (Fig. 11) and the *olfactory tract.* Numerous sensory fibers extend from the olfactory bulb through the *lamina cribrosa* (sieve—like membrane) at the base of the skull to the nasal cavity (the fibers are indicated in Fig. 10). Hypophysis and Pituitary are synonymous terms. The ventricle of the olfactory system does not exist in man and therefore is not indicated; in animals, it extends from the olfactory bulb through the olfactory tract to the lateral ventricle.

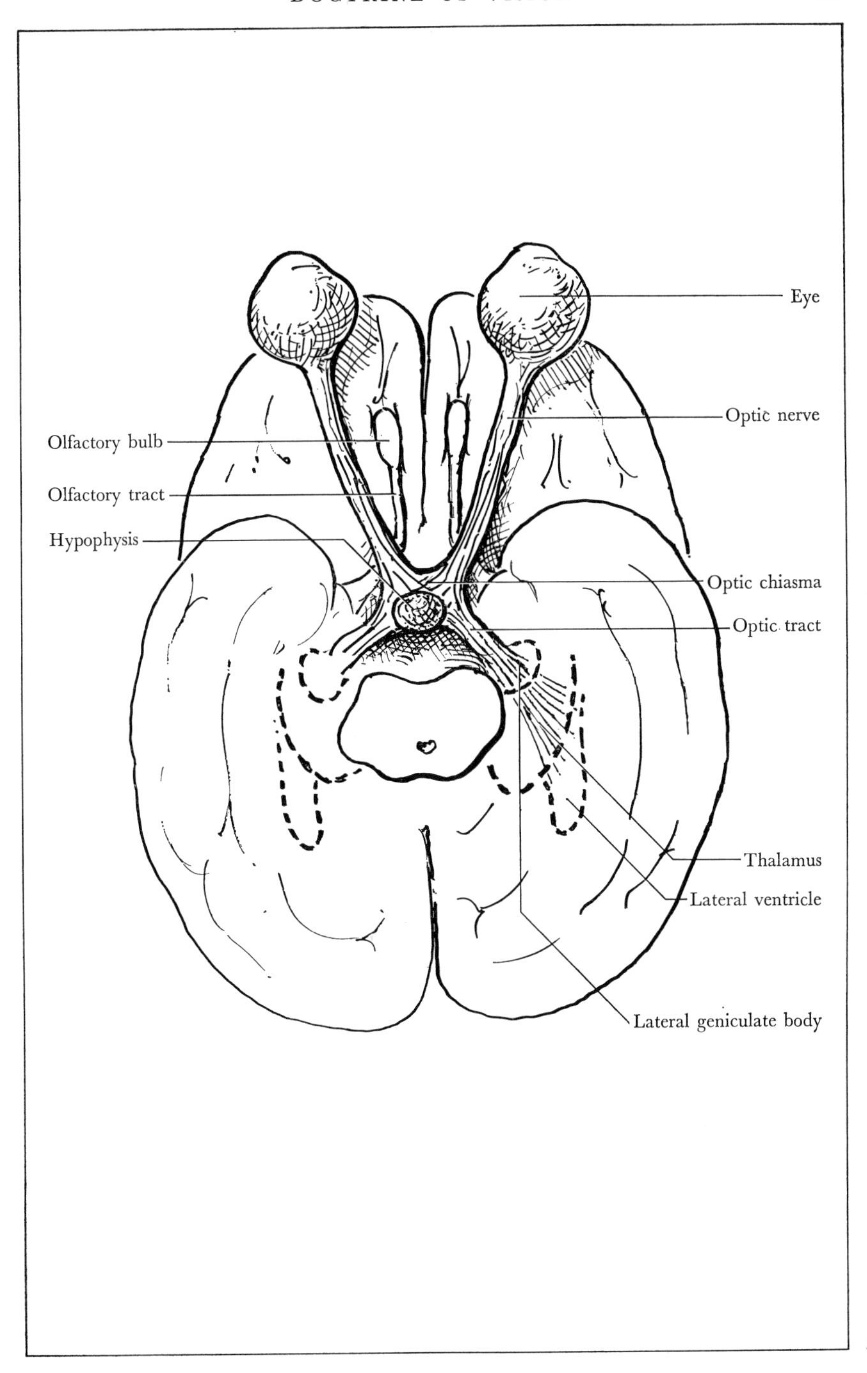
Eye
Optic nerve
Olfactory bulb
Olfactory tract
Hypophysis
Optic chiasma
Optic tract
Thalamus
Lateral ventricle
Lateral geniculate body

ly, as if to show simply and solely that they only came in contact in order to unite their canals.' [139]

Galen did not realize that the optic nerve was composed of individual fibers, although he noticed that the optic nerve spread out into fibers composing the retina, after it had entered the eyes. He assumed that a complete fusion of the two optic canals takes place at the crossing. This erroneous idea had originated with ALCMAEON of Croton in the early 5th century B.C. Modern anatomical studies demonstrated, however, that only a small central blood vessel is visible in the part of the optic nerve nearest the eyeball. Galen even wrote that the upper opening of the canal into the ventricles is hardly visible. In repeating Galen's dissection of the ox-eye, I could not find a central vein in the optic nerve, which appeared solid in its entire course, although Galen stated that he could probe this canal with a fine hog bristle [138]. However, these eyes were bloodless, whereas Galen had stressed the importance of using eyes with congested veins.

Since Galen remained undecided whether the cerebral pneuma was flowing back and forth through the optic nerve, he did not state

139 SHASTID, p. 8612 (1911); KUEHN, vol. 3, p. 814.—*Epallatesthai* means both: to become intermixed and to cross; the context makes the latter translation more acceptable.

Figure 4. Galen's concept of the relation between the optic nerves and the cerebral ventricles (lateral view; schematic drawing).

According to Galen the optic nerves continue after the crossing at the chiasma and terminate at a part of the lateral ventricles which he called the *thalamus* (i.e. chamber). Galen did not describe the optic fibers past the *chiasma* as optic tract as we do. In distinction to Galen's terminology, the modern expression *thalamus* corresponds to a body of ganglia on the base of the lateral ventricle which is indicated as a shaded area. According to Galen the lateral ventricles communicate with the 3rd ventricle and drain residual phlegm from there through the infundibulum (i.e. funnel) and the pituitary gland into the nasal cavity. Posteriorly the 3rd ventricle extends into the 4th ventricle. This junction was thought to be rhythmically opened or closed by rocking motions of the cerebellum, esp. the vermis cerebelli (SIEGEL, p. 122, 1968). This mechanism supposedly controlled the flow of cerebral pneuma *(spiritus animalis)*. Abbreviations: III.V.: 3rd ventricle; IV.V.: 4th ventricle; V.V.: 5th ventricle of the brain.

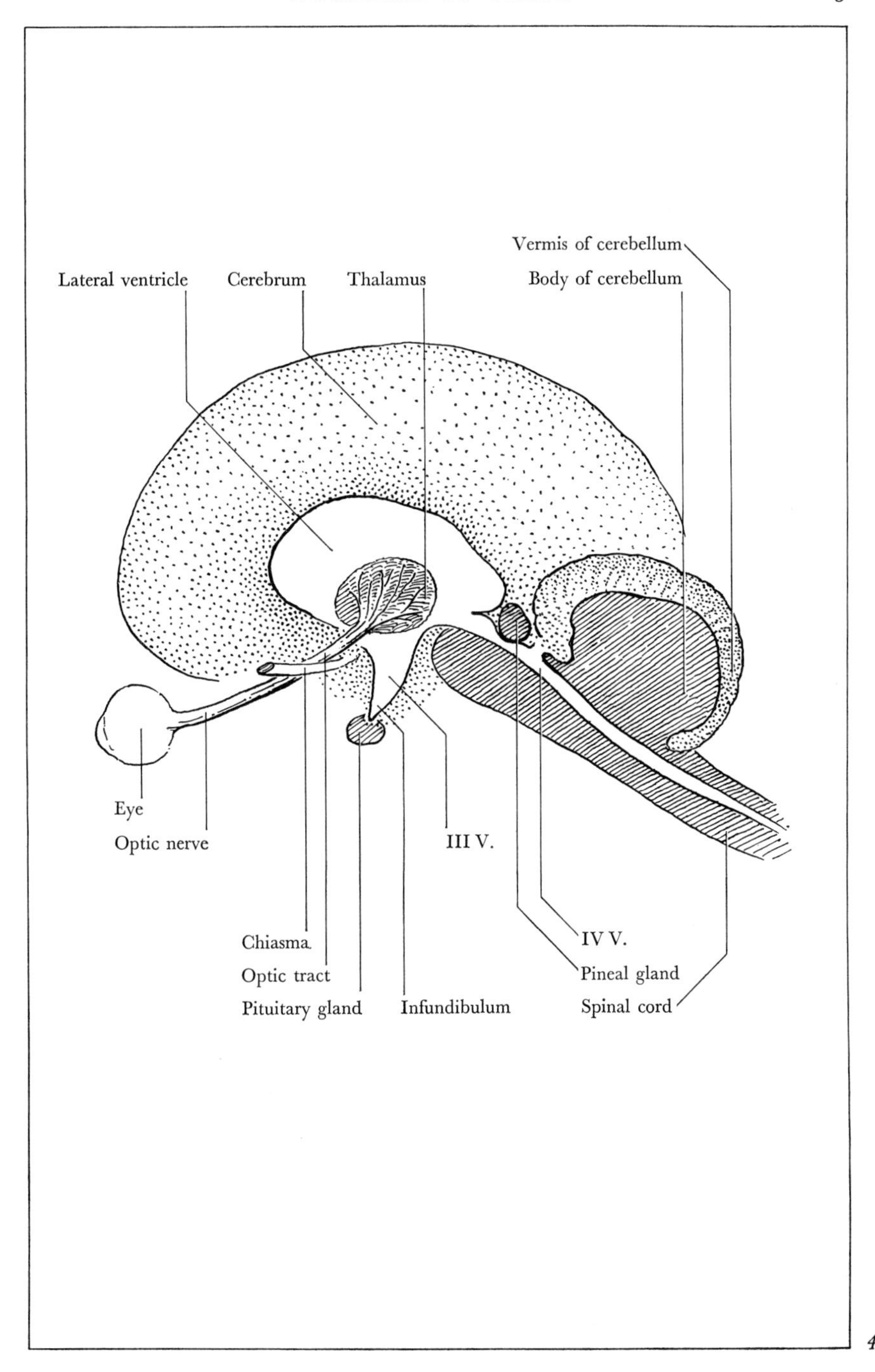
Vermis of cerebellum
Lateral ventricle
Cerebrum
Thalamus
Body of cerebellum
Eye
Optic nerve
III V.
Chiasma
Optic tract
Pituitary gland
Infundibulum
IV V.
Pineal gland
Spinal cord

whether it passed outside along the optic nerve or through its central canal *(poros)*. He only wrote:

> 'One part of the brain extends itself until it reaches the lens (literally, the crystalline humor) in order to recognize the impressions *(gnosis ton pathematon)* [which the lens receives]. It stands to reason that this extension includes a sensory conduit *(poros)*, because only thus can it enclose an abundance of cerebral pneuma.'[140]

Whatever the details of this doctrine may have been, Galen outlined a two-way movement of the pneuma through both retina and optic nerve: first from the brain through optic nerve and retina to the lens and further into space toward the object of vision; then backward to the eye, carrying the visual perception to the brain (see also p. 54).

Galen thought that after the loss of one eye the vision of the remaining eye was enhanced, since under normal conditions the cerebral pneuma was flowing from the brain to both eyes through the interconnection of both optic nerves at their crossing, the *chiasma* (see Fig. 3). He drew from observation the faulty conclusion that we can see better with one eye when we close the other eye, since pneuma flows in larger quantities via the chiasma to the active eye[141].

Galen did not suspect, nor did he have methods of determining, that the optic tract leads ultimately not into the ventricle but into the occipital lobe of the brain. Prejudiced by the thought that the pneuma occupied the cerebral ventricles as the 'organ' of all mental functions, he erroneously deduced from dissection that the optic nerves terminated at the lateral ventricles. Galen wrote that it would have impressed him as more logical if both optic nerves would have arisen from one single area of the brain. Such an arrangement, he reasoned, might have improved the understanding of visual perception, since then we would deal only with one common receptacle of sensation'[142].

140 DAREMBERG, vol. 1, p. 544; KUEHN, vol. 3, pp. 641–642. Galen explained cataract erroneously as blockage of these passages; KUEHN, vol. 5, p. 635.

141 KUEHN, vol. 5, p. 614; vol. 3, p. 836; Galen, *De usu partium*, book 10, chap. 14. The latter comparison disregards that we see better stereoscopically; see also p. 106.

142 The idea of a single center of perception reflects ARISTOTLE's concept of the *sensus communis*. This idea, combined with a doctrine of vision, was the erroneous basis of DESCARTES' doctrine of the role of the pineal gland in visual perception.

Anatomical studies suggested to Galen that the optic nerves could also serve as a possible conduit of light rays to the cerebral ventricles, the seat of visual perception. Since Galen described that each optic nerve entered the eyeball at a point exactly opposite to the center of the cornea, he thought that the central ray (optical axis) could pass straight through the center of the cornea and lens to the optic nerve[235]. He had failed to recognize that the optical axis meets the background of the eye at a point slightly lateral of the point (optic disc) where the optic nerve enters the eyeball. The narrow area where the visual axis hits the retina is known today as the area of maximal vision *(macula)*. However, Galen based a second, the geometrical, doctrine of vision, on an anatomical error, in the belief that the light rays entering the optic nerve at the optic disc continue their rectilinear passage through the optic nerve. This error of observation was the principal justification of Galen's second doctrine of vision (p. 86ff.).

e) Pupillary Movement, a Pneumatic Mechanism (Figure 5)

Galen attributed to the outgoing stream of pneuma still another function: the regulation of the size of the pupillary aperture by inflating or deflating the iris around the pupil. The latter effect seemed only to be possible if the pneuma had a measurable mass or volume. But according to Galen and the Stoic writers the cerebral pneuma was an invisible and weightless agent. Likewise, when Galen spoke of the conduction of the optical image, he did not attribute to the pneuma the physical properties of air. For our understanding, however, a pneuma responsible for the movement of the pupil would need the material features of what we define as gas. Galen's twofold usage of the term 'pneuma' cannot be overlooked, since his idea of the cerebral pneuma as an assumed agent of greatest subtlety contradicted his concept that the cavities (ventricles) of the brain were filled with an air-like pneuma[143]. But Galen had evidently a spacefilling agent in mind when he spoke of the regulation of the pupillary movements. This doctrine was based on painstaking observations.

Galen correctly described the anterior chamber of the eye between

143 Discussed in the chapter on nerve action: SIEGEL, p. 113ff. (1968), and in this book on p. 46, 47.

cornea and lens and likewise the posterior chamber, 'the space between iris and lens'[144]. He observed that the chambers are filled with a clear fluid which escapes after removal of the deepest layer of the cornea[145]. He assumed that some cerebral pneuma penetrated unnoticed into this watery humor, entering from the terminal endings of the retinal fibers. It was the same pneuma which he also declared responsible for dilating the pupil by inflating the iris through its retinal attachments.

Galen likened the iris to an elastic circular tube. He thought that the deflated iris appeared flat with a narrow opening in the middle; but that if it expanded its volume on inflation it simultaneously retracted its inner margin. Thus, inflation by the pneuma would enlarge the pupil, whereas deflation of the iris would narrow the pupillary aperture (see Fig. 5).

Galen's description of this mechanism of pupillary movement has so far not been discussed in the literature, although it is of historical interest, since a similar mechanism of muscular movement by inflation with pneuma was proposed by later philosophers such as DESCARTES (p. 70). Contrary to the opinion of some authors, Galen's text does not suggest that only an increased amount of pneuma in the chamber of the eye, i.e. inside the opening of the pupil, pushes the inner margin of the pupil outward and enlarges the pupil. He stated that the pneuma in the iris itself is responsible for the pupillary movement, although he considered that variation of the amount of fluid and pneuma in the pupillary space could also affect the position of iris and uvea and, in this manner, the size of the pupil itself.

144 DUCKWORTH, p. 37.
145 DUCKWORTH, p. 37; also DAREMBERG, vol. 1, p. 621; Galen, *De usu partium*, book 10, chap. 5; KUEHN, vol. 3, p. 781.

Figure 5. Galen's concept of the mechanism of pupillary movements.

Galen believed that the *pupil* is dilated, when both the *iris* and *uvea* are inflated (i.e. full), but that the pupil becomes narrow ('contracted'), when both are emptied of pneuma. He thought that the *cerebral pneuma (spiritus animalis)* entered the iris from the optic nerves via the retina and the uvea (which is attached to the retina; see also Fig. 1). He did not know that the smooth muscles and nerve fibers of the iris and uvea constitute the mechanism of pupillary contraction. Uvea and ciliary body are synonymous terms. The term uvea illustrates the 'grape' like protrusions at the posterior wall of the iris.

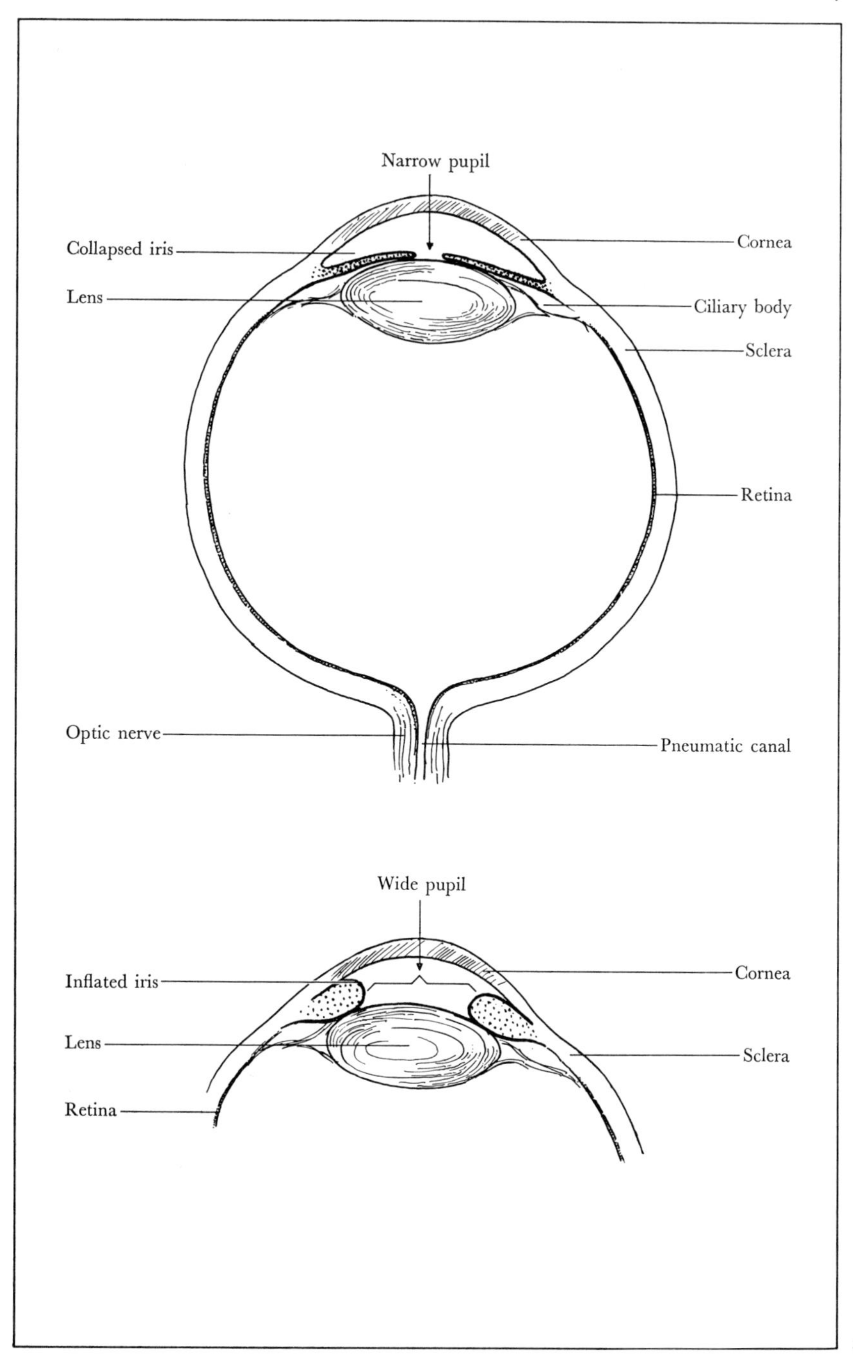
Narrow pupil
Collapsed iris
Cornea
Lens
Ciliary body
Sclera
Retina
Optic nerve
Pneumatic canal
Wide pupil
Inflated iris
Cornea
Lens
Sclera
Retina

5

The following quotation suggests that Galen even undertook experiments to prove his pneumatic doctrine of pupillary movements. He evidently introduced a thin hollow probe through the external coats of the eye into the uvea which he inflated by blowing air through this tube. Referring to the idea that an increased flow of pneuma into the uvea caused enlargement of the pupil *(mydriasis)* he wrote:

> 'It is obvious to reason that the pupil becomes thus enlarged; but you can try by artificial preparation and experiment *(di' epitechneseos . . . kai basanisais)* to verify what is obviously apparent *(autois tois enargos phainomenois)*. If you inflate the iris with air *(pneuma)* from inside you will see that the opening of the pupil dilates. Experience proves therefore that the pupil becomes enlarged, because [the iris] is filled with pneuma. Further, this statement does not imply more than that the iris, when inflated internally, expands and distends considerably, but that in this fashion the [pupillary] opening becomes enlarged. The same happens when other bodies of membranous substance and delicate structure retract into themselves.' [146]

It was tempting to repeat these experiments. But I obtained the opposite results. First, I incised the center of the cornea in order to be able to remove the cornea along the corneo-scleral border without injury to the iris. The iris faced us now and air was injected by a narrow needle. Because air escaped too easily I used water. However, I observed only a considerable narrowing of the pupil after two or three different areas of the iris had been injected. The iris does not rise like a tire, and when it gains in volume the pupil 'contracts'. The same result can be obtained when one opens the eye from the rear. After radially incising the sclera, starting at the entrance of the optic nerve, one extrudes carefully vitreous, iris and lens together. Then, one can inflate the iris with water. Again it was apparent that the pupillary opening became narrower when the iris was 'inflated'. These experiments are quite difficult because of the fragility of the iris and the post-mortem narrowing of the pupil of the ox-eye. This outcome seemed to contradict Galen's results.

Furthermore, Galen reasoned that inflation of the pupil by pneuma had to be so rapid that a fluid agent could hardly be held responsible

146 Daremberg, vol. 1, p. 621; Kuehn, vol. 3, pp. 782–783.

for the pupillary movement. Also, when one eye is closed rapid diversion only of a subtle pneuma to the other eye could instantly dilate the pupil of the other eye[147]. An exception, he thought, occurred in disease of the eyeball when the flow of pneuma through the optic nerve was obstructed (i.e. through the assumed central canal of this nerve, see p. 59). We can assert that Galen's observation of the enlargement of the contralateral pupil after closure of the other eye was indeed correct. It also offered him an additional argument in favor of his pneumatic concept of pupillary motion.

Galen raised the question whether we can truly believe that cerebral pneuma could flow into the iris through connecting fibers of the retina, since these delicate structures could only be seen with great difficulty. He mentioned these doubts, although in another context he had described the apparently more plainly visible connections between iris and retina (Fig. 2), the radially arranged spokes of the uveal (ciliary) body. We read:

> 'We must ask, since indeed the pneuma travels to the eye through [the pores of] the optic nerve and equally through all other nerves, whether its path is invisible because they are so narrow, or whether it appears impossible, since there are only the very finest fibers in the nerves.'[148]

Since he apparently still had some doubts about the agent responsible for pupillary motion, he described its effect as a hydraulic mechanism, without reference to pneuma:

> 'When the choroid membrane including the [posterior wall of the] iris *(rhagoeides chiton, uvea)* is distended by some matter *(ousia)* which fills it up, the pupil becomes dilated.'[149]

By employing the term *ousia* Galen simply indicated 'matter' without specifying its composition.

147 KUEHN, vol. 5, p. 614.—Galen overlooked that the pupil is completely distended after death when, according to his doctrine, the pneuma should have left the eye. There is no reference in his writings to this observation which completely contradicts his doctrine of pupillary movement.

148 KUEHN, vol. 5, p. 616.

149 KUEHN, vol. 5, p. 614.

Galen's concept of a pneumatic mechanism of pupillary motion seemed to be supported by the observation that frequently the pupils of old people became very narrow. He thought that the tissues of the cornea and iris dry up and shrivel, because the body contained less pneuma with advancing age. We do observe in many old people very narrow, almost pinpoint-sized pupils, but for reasons other than those Galen assumed.

Galen advanced the concept of a pneumatic mechanism of the pupillary motion, since he was not aware of the presence of muscle fibers or nerves in the pupil. However, Galen's doctrine of the contraction of the skeletal muscle was contrary to his explanation of the movement of the pupil. First he thought muscular contractions of the skeletal muscles were initiated either by a quality or force *(dynamis)* passing along the nerve or by a pneuma traveling through a canal in the nerve. He even called the peripheral nerves waterpipes *(ochetoi)*, which would favor the concept of a space-occupying pneuma, as in the case of the iris. However, Galen tried but failed to demonstrate the hypothetical channels for the transport of pneuma through the peripheral nerves to the skeletal muscles. Therefore, the concept of muscle innervation by the progression of a contractile force along the peripheral nerve appeared to him more likely[150].

Galen's pneumatic doctrine might have been of influence on DESCARTES who thought that all nerves were hollow ducts conducting air. But DESCARTES postulated that delicate channels in all nerves were equipped with valves which could maintain a one-way flow of pneuma. This would allow a separate flow either to the brain in the sensory nerves or to the periphery via the motor nerves. It is difficult to decide whether DESCARTES was influenced by Galen's concept of a pneumatic control of the pupillary motion, since he never quoted Galen, or whether he knew a similar inflation doctrine of the muscle by ERASISTRATUS whom Galen opposed (KUEHN, vol. 8, p. 429), or whether he modified doctrines of his own contemporaries.

150 In regard to the innervation of the skeletal muscles: DAREMBERG, vol. 2, p. 323; KUEHN, vol. 4, p. 371. About the motion of the pupils: see DAREMBERG, vol. 1, p. 621; KUEHN, vol. 3, p. 783. Often Galen remained ambiguous about the employment of the term *dynamis* and *pneuma*; but we have always to check the Greek text, since DAREMBERG, for instance, translated *pege* as 'channel', although it indicated only the 'source' of the dynamis (loc. cit.); KUEHN, vol. 4, p. 371. More details in SIEGEL, p. 183 (1968).

f) Principles of Pneumatic Transmission of the Optic Image

We discussed in the last chapter on pupillary control the effect of a pneuma, presumably of a material, space-occupying nature. In the present chapter, we will deal with the other aspect of Galen's concept of pneuma, to which a specific neurological or physiological function was attributed. It was the type of pneuma which often was identified with *dynamis*, force. This type of pneuma was related to the qualities, it was regarded as spatially extended but not of tangible nature.

It has already been brought out that Galen distinguished three phases of visual perception by pneuma: sensitization of the space for optical transmission by pneuma; reception of the incoming image by the cerebral pneuma in the eye; and conduction of the pneuma carrying the image to the brain. It is difficult to understand that the ancient philosophers could accept the idea that an emanation of cerebral pneuma into space meets the incoming image. This could only occur after the eye had already been directed toward the object. If the doctrine of an outgoing emanation was correct, then the act of visual perception must be preceded by an act of awareness of the same object, unless it relied on chance. This paradox appears as the prime obstacle to our understanding of the pneumatic doctrine of vision, whether we talk of PLATO, of the Stoics or of Galen himself.

The importance of awareness for Galen's doctrine of vision has to be understood as the result of the psychological orientation of the ancient philosophers in regard to the problems of perception. The concept of an outward stream of pneuma had its roots in the ideas of PLATO and EMPEDOCLES[151], who were probably under the impression that they had identified a physical event. Likewise, EUCLID's explanation of the fact that we often do not perceive a small object unless we look for it specifically[152] was psychologically oriented (see p. 14).

The ancient idea that an outgoing emanation traveled from the observer's eye toward the object of vision was also compatible with the materialistic concept of the ancient philosophers about the soul. Since they regarded the mind as a material agent they had no reason for differentiating clearly the psychological function from the physiological reaction of the cerebral pneuma.

151 See p. 16, 23.
152 VER EECKE, p. 2: proposition I.

Based on this tradition, Galen pictured the cerebral pneuma as a mediator or carrier of mental function which was not only present in the substance of the brain and its cavities but could also extend its activity into space [153]. (The injured brain supposedly lost all its sensory, motor and psychic functions by escape of the cerebral pneuma.) Galen related visual perception to an active state of the cerebral pneuma present simultaneously in space, in the eye and in the optic nerve. It was not as difficult for Galen, as it may apear to us, to postulate that pneuma could extend its influence beyond the limits of the eye. The travel through the space and the interaction of the pneuma with the spacefilling medium (regardless of whether it was air or another medium) remained in agreement with Galen's general physiological doctrine which was based on the concept of qualities. He wrote:

> 'The qualitative change *(alloiosis)* induced by the incoming picture is transmitted to the central sense organ [i.e. the brain, *tes psyches hegemonikon*]' [154] [since it contains a perceptive faculty].
>
> 'Sensation is not the qualitative change as such, but it is the recognition of this change *(diagnosis tes alloioseos)*.' [155]

The doctrine of these qualitative changes *(alloiosis)* of pneuma, resulting from contact with the object, requires some further explanation. [156]

All substances which constitute the living body were supposedly composed of a substrate *(soma, ousia)* and various qualities. External stimuli effected an increase, decrease or transfer of these qualities. This concept formed the basis of Galen's biological doctrine and especially of his interpretation of sense perception. Changes which we would define as physical, chemical or physiological were explained as result of an exchange, loss or gain of qualities *(alloiosis)*. We are aware today that this doctrine was erroneous, since the concept of qualities was only derived from sense perception, whereas the ancients presumed that they actually existed independently in the surrounding world.

Galen spoke frequently of qualities which were not as well defined

153 SIEGEL, pp. 113, 119 (1968) discussed the production of *cerebral pneuma (spiritus animalis)*.

154 KUEHN, vol. 5, p. 641.

155 KUEHN, vol. 5, p. 636.

156 For more details, see SIEGEL, p. 183–195 (1968).

as the four basic qualities of hot, cold, dry and moist[157]. For example, he described that fishermen, after touching a torpedo fish with a harpoon, often suffered pain, coma or temporary paralysis of a limb because of the transfer of a certain powerful quality from the fish through the harpoon into the body[158]. The 'narcotic effect' of the electric discharge of the torpedo fish was explained as the transfer of this unknown quality. Galen did not attach to it a name nor did he call it 'electricity', but compared it with the narcotic quality *(poiotes)* or effect *(dynamis)* of certain drugs. Even magnetism[159] was included into this conceptual system, since the attracting power of a magnet was regarded as an undefined 'quality' drawing the iron through the intervening space[160]. Galen thought of these 'qualities' when he formulated his doctrine of visual transmission.

In the framework of these ideas certain qualities inherent to the pneuma were assumed to exert their influence beyond the confines of the eyeball. In other words, it appeared quite conceivable to Galen that the pneuma induced qualitative changes *(alloiosis)* in the medium which occupied the space in front of the eye. It is of importance for this interpretation to understand that this effect of pneuma did not postulate the transmission of a corpuscular agent. Galen's pneumatic agent of vision had this similarity to ARISTOTLE's luminous ether-like medium: a qualitative change traveling through a stationary medium.

Galen's pneumatic doctrine of visual perception may be illustrated by referring to the results of recent research on the space-perception of certain fish, which perceive distant objects by modifications of an electric field. These fish constantly emit this field from an electric organ located in the tailfin:

> 'Electric receptors of certain fish ... can detect obstacles at sunless depth ... These fish emit pulses of low voltage with frequencies

157 See SIEGEL, p. 145 (1968) were full references are given. A good survey is presented by Galen in the treatise *On the natural faculties* (Engl. transl., see BROCK [1952], book 1, chap. 2).

158 KUEHN, vol. 8, p. 72; vol. 7, p. 109.

159 KUEHN, vol. 2, pp. 45–48; KUEHN, vol. 8, p. 422.

160 The relation between the concept of qualities and modern chemical concepts has been discussed in SIEGEL, p. 148 (1968), with regard to the problem of mixture and fusion, which in turn is related to the question of ultimate particles and infinite divisibility. This was discussed recently by HORNE (1966) and SAMBURSKI, p. 143 ff. (1956).

characteristic of each species. The change of the pattern of the electric field as the result of objects ... in the surrounding water is detected [by sensory cells in the skin of the fish]. They can even tell when someone approaches the aquarium carrying a small stationary magnet.'[161]

Although emission and perception of electromagnetic changes is not mediated by the eye of this fish, the pattern of its sense perception appears comparable to the Galenic doctrine of pneuma; it represents a model for Galen's pneumatic concept of vision, since the emitted waves rebound from objects in front of the fish like Galen's pneuma which supposedly returns from the object of vision.

The fish even senses 'lines of orientation', although a diffuse electric field surrounds its body. This observation reminds one of the uncertainty in Galen's doctrine of vision as to whether a diffuse pneuma or rectilinear light rays had to be considered as basis of visual perception. It has to be stressed, however, that the Galenic doctrine of sense perception was based on anatomical observations interpreted in the light of philosophical concepts, whereas the field-doctrine of electric perception by fish is based on experimental methods. In spite of a certain similarity of concepts a true comparison is not possible between results of Galen's deductive and modern inductive reasoning.

Galen undoubtedly considered the pneuma as a physical agent, since he regarded the cerebral pneuma only as 'organ of the soul' even though the material nature of the pneuma remained undefined[162]. He refused to identify pneuma and soul, the nature of which he did not want to discuss in a medical treatise.

It is important to realize that Galen did not recognize a specific visual pneuma. He did not accept the Stoic idea of a specialization of the cerebral pneuma into subqualities such as a separate visual or auditory pneuma. Although the Stoic philosophers wrote that each type of sense perception was mediated by a specific pneuma[163], Galen believed that only a single type of cerebral pneuma existed which acted locally according to the special structure of each sense organ[164]. Galen

161 CARR, p. 32 (1967); LISSMANN (1958); LISSMANN and MACHIN (1958).
162 KUEHN, vol. 5, p. 645; vol. 4, pp. 501–502: 'The brain is the principal seat of sensation and of active motion.' For other references: SIEGEL, pp. 192, 193 (1968).
163 ARNOLD, pp. 245–250.
164 SIEGEL, pp. 183ff. (1968).

clearly stated that the action of the cerebral pneuma in the eye could produce only visual perception, whereas the same pneuma served other sense perceptions in other organs. This was an anticipation of JOHANNES VON MUELLER'S (1801–1858) concept of the specificity of sense perception [165].

Fully aware that the assumed pneumatic emanation from the eye alone appeared insufficient to explain visual perception, Galen did not fail to relate the perception of an optical image to the simultaneous action of sunlight in a manner which reminds us of PLATO (p. 25):

> 'The surrounding air becomes apparently modified likewise by both the extension of the [cerebral] pneuma and by the luminosity of the sun. The latter, by getting in contact with it from above, communicates its whole power. The [mechanism of] vision through the optic nerve is essentially [based] on the pneuma: when it touches the surrounding [medium] *(to periechonti)*, and at its first contact with it the pneuma produces an alteration *(alloiosis)* which it communicates to the utmost [confines of space] . . . This alteration pervades in the shortest time the entire space. We consider it likewise as an effect of the innate power *(dynamis)* of the sun . . . The surrounding air and the nerves have some similarity of their substance *(physis)* according to their composition.' [166]

Galen recognized that the transmission of light was different from the transmission of heat or cold, since the latter required a specific carrier. He wrote:

> 'In vision, eye and air are simultaneously affected and the alteration ceases instantly with the disappearance of the luminous body. However, heat or cold remain after the radiating body has been removed.' [167]

Since Galen regarded either pneuma or light separately as insufficient for visual perception, he postulated the fusion of both as in-

165 GARRISON, p. 452.
166 KUEHN, vol. 5, pp. 619–620. The last sentence of this quotation refers to their susceptibility to *alloiosis*, i.e. to qualitative change.
167 KUEHN, vol. 5, p. 620 (condensed).

dispensable: the cerebral pneuma, meeting the sunlight on the surface of the object of vision, was transformed into an activated state[168].

An additional difficulty of Galen's pneumatic doctrine of vision arose from his failure to explain the transmission of an orderly picture from the lens to the cerebral ventricles. Galen acknowledged the formation of a consistent image of the object of vision at the anterior surface of the lens. But he remained silent about the problem of how an optically consistent transfer of this image could take place by the pneuma, firstly through the fibrous connections from lens to retina, secondly through the central canal of the optic nerve and the chiasma (where both streams meet) into the ventricles. A point-to-point transmission of the image appeared evidently impossible by a flow of pneuma, but equal difficulties were posed by the geometrical doctrine of vision (see p. 86), since all rectilinear rays were thought to enter the narrow optic canal for further propagation to the cerebral ventricles. The silence of the ancient scientists on this point was reflected by a similar disregard of this logical problem by medieval scientists.

g) Synopsis of Galen's Pneumatic Doctrine of Vision

The following quotations will recapitulate Galen's pneumatic doctrine of vision in his own words:

> 'In regard to the object of vision *(blepomenon)* there are two possibilities: either that it emits something *(ti)* from itself[169] by which it will initiate its own recognition or, if it should not emit anything, one could expect that some sensory power *(dynamis)* arrives there from us. Which of both alternatives is more correct has first to be decided.'[170]

Without mentioning ARISTOTLE's transparent medium Galen explained:

168 The Stoics postulated a combination of light with pneuma, whereas ARISTOTLE spoke of the activation of the transparent medium by light through *alloiosis*; KUEHN, vol. 5, p. 643.

169 Galen refuted the possibility of a spontaneous emission from the object to the eye as unlikely. KUEHN, vol. 5, p. 618.

170 KUEHN, vol. 5, p. 618; further discussion in KUEHN, vol. 5, p. 617.

'The question arises whether something travels to us in some manner from the object which we see, or whether the air serves as instrument for visual perception, comparable to the nerves which mediate perception through touch . . . The [optic] nerve is part of the brain, like a branch or part of a tree, and takes up a power for recognition of that which it touches. The air around us is transformed into a compatible condition; when it is illuminated by the sun it becomes an instrument of vision equally to the cerebral pneuma. But before it has been illuminated, it cannot be considered as rendered a sensory instrument only by the impact of the cerebral pneuma.' [171]

Obviously the problem was so difficult that Galen did not have a definite answer to the question of whether air or another agent carried the optic image through space. Since he was reluctant to give a final opinion about the physical nature of the visual transmission through space, he occasionally used the term the 'surrounding' instead of air:

'It appears likely that the pneuma arriving in the eye [from the brain] unites itself instantly with the surrounding *(periechonti)* and alters it, according to its own nature, but it does not extend itself over a great distance.' [172]

'Its distribution produces a qualitative change in manner similar to the sunrays which likewise affect the air.' ' From this it follows that the surrounding air serves us as a [sensory] organ during the time of vision like the nerves in the entire body.' [173]

Galen linked the 'escape' of cerebral pneuma into space *(ekptosis)* to the effect of the sunrays which render space fit for optical transmission.

The concept of 'air' as used by Galen needs some clarification. Galen stated that the visual pneuma 'assimilated' itself to the 'air' surrounding the eye, whereas by hearing or smelling we perceive changes of the 'air' in another purely mechanical manner. Obviously 'air' had

171 KUEHN, vol. 5, pp. 641–642. 'Power' in Greek is *dynamis*, indicating the transfer of a quality from the object to the nerve or sense organ (see p. 47, 70).
172 KUEHN, vol. 5, p. 617.
173 KUEHN, vol. 5, p. 619 (slightly arranged).

several meanings. After a discussion of the various interpretations of this term by the philosophers Galen came to the conclusion:

> 'We adhere to the opinion that air *(aer)* is a basic substance, continuous in itself and nowhere interwoven by empty space.'[174]
>
> 'But the substance *(ousia)* of air *(aer)* which we smell consists of thicker parts than the luminous *(auge)*[175] [air]; likewise the vapor *(atmos)* which we [breathe] is again thicker than the air *(aer)* [which we smell].'[176]

Each sense organ appeared to be adapted to a different quality of 'air': the eye perceived the luminous *(augoeides)*, the ear the airlike *(aeroeides)* and the nose the vaporous *(atmoeides)* characteristic of the air[177]. Galen did not distinguish the different physical components of the air as we do but evidently spoke of different 'airs' according to the different types of sense perception. This interpretation of the term air is in agreement with RONCHI's analysis that the terms of ancient 'physics' corresponded more to the modern ideas about psychology of sense perception than to our physical concepts. The Greeks had discovered some laws of perception, form and color, but their 'optics' were not a chapter of physics[178].

h) Luminescence

Galen's discussion of luminescence gives us further insight into the reasons for his misunderstanding the true nature of light and visual perception. If he had grasped the importance of luminescence, he most likely would have abandoned the idea that visual perception depended essentially on the emanation of pneuma from the eye.

ARISTOTLE had already referred to vision without sunlight. Galen wrote that a luminous emanation from the eye of some animals such as lions and leopards activates the transparent medium. He considered,

174 KUEHN, vol. 8, p. 673; i.e. continuous but not corpuscular.
175 Galen seemed to use the term *auge* for a transmitted light without indicating a known light-source.
176 KUEHN, vol. 7, p. 122.
177 KUEHN, vol. 5, p. 627; KUEHN, vol. 2, pp. 862, 864.
178 RONCHI, pp. 12, 19, 20 (1957).

however, this biological source of light only as a substitute for sunlight during darkness[179]. ARISTOTLE had stated this in more detail than Galen:

> 'Not everything is visible in the light [of the sun] but only the proper color of each thing. Some things, however, are not seen in light but cause perception *(poiei aisthesin)* in the dark, such as those which appear fiery or luminous (there is no single expression for these), like fungi, flesh, or the heads, scales and eyes of fishes. In none of these is a proper color seen. But such things are visible for another reason.'[180]

ARISTOTLE believed that color was due to a reflection of the sunlight from the surface of the objects, but not an essential factor of the light itself. Luminescent animals, therefore, were thought to emit a neutral light[181] from their own body but not color, since reflection was not involved.

Galen mentioned only briefly the observations of phosphorescence in his treatise on vision, without referring to the question of color. He said:

> 'Thick and gleaming is the skin of these animals. Because of this light *(selas)* some have been called *selachii*.'[182]

Galen mentioned that this type of light was also characteristic of the firefly, the glowworm, the lantern fish and some other luminescent animals, of rotten wood, of sea-water and the sea shore where, as we know today, it arises from the growth of certain bacteria and fungi. Electrical phenomena of the aurora borealis and St. Elmo's fire on the masts of ships also were erroneously regarded as spontaneous luminescence[183].

These phenomena did not contradict Galen's pneumatic doctrine of vision, but rather furnished him with additional support for this

179 KUEHN, vol. 5, p. 616.
180 ARISTOTLE, *On the soul*, II, 7: 419 a 1–10 (slightly modified).
181 See chapter on color, p. 82.
182 KUEHN, vol. 6, p. 737; the name *selachii* is still currently used as the zoological term for sharks and related species.
183 HARVEY, p. 43 (1957).

doctrine. Since Galen thought that the 'light' issuing from the eyes of lions and panthers in darkness enabled these animals to perceive during the night, he promptly attributed the luminous radiation to a pneuma emitted by their eyes[184]. This appears as a rather strange statement, in view of Galen's postulate that the pneuma issuing from the eyes had to fuse with external light (p. 77).

Galen did not discuss whether luminous bodies emitted a diffuse light or distinct light rays. Since the light from luminescent organs seemed to belong to the category of pneumatic emanations, he did not even consider whether or not it was composed of light rays. Had Galen experimented more extensively with artificial light, he might have even recognized that the rules of light rays could equally be applied to the behavior of luminescent light. But he was too deeply indoctrinated with the pneumatic idea to consider this type of vision as independent of the cerebral pneuma.

i) Day-Blindness (Hemeralopy)

Galen wrote that he often noticed that intense sunlight could overpower the weak light which the eyes supposedly emitted. This conflict was thought to lead to the suppression of the weaker light-source. Thus, he observed that we cannot perceive a weak light near a strong source of light, or that the eye is temporarily or permanently blinded by too strong an illumination.

Galen noted also that we can perceive stars during the daytime when looking up from a deep well, provided that the sun is not in the zenith; likewise, that some stars become visible during eclipse of the sun; also that the light of a candle seems to disappear in full daylight. He wrote:

> 'You will see how a lamp-light fades at once when placed in the sun.'[185]

184 KUEHN, vol. 5, p. 616. Galen spoke of a visual cone formed by the light emanating from the eyes of these animals at night. But the assumption of an optical cone does not suggest whether we are dealing with a continuous pneumatic stream of light or with distinct light rays.

185 KUEHN, vol. 3, p. 777.

'The weaker [light] is always overcome and dispersed by the stronger one.' [186]

'The power of sight is injured by a strong and shining light.' [187]

He thought that this conflict occurred in the eyeball itself, i.e. in pupil, lens or vitreous, where both the outgoing and incoming light 'communicate and mix' *(koinonia kai krasis)* [188]. Galen did not recognize the principle of fatigue or contrast as the reason for this effect.

Galen explained by the same assumption the permanent damage of the eye from overexposure to very strong illumination. He wrote that the visual emanation of the eye and therefore the 'power of vision' could be permanently abolished by a strong external light. He cited some interesting observations to prove his point: the soldiers of XENOPHON's army became completely blinded on their march through the snow fields of Asia Minor from exposure to the intense reflection [189]. He told another story about the tyrant DIONYSUS of Sicily who diabolically rejoiced in punishing his prisoners by blinding them: he fitted above their dungeon a small chamber, perfectly whitewashed, with large windows facing the sun. After long confinement in dark chambers he led his victims to this brightly illuminated room. Looking into this splendor with great joy, they soon became completely blinded, since their eyes could not tolerate the sudden exposure [190]. Galen also mentioned that copyists who had to write on white parchment for long periods of time, used to interrupt their tedious work frequently in order to look at colored objects lest their visual power suffer [190]. It appeared to Galen, therefore, as a foregone conclusion that 'the light of the eyes can be destroyed' by strong illumination. Galen also mentioned that many people who tried to observe the solar eclipse with unprotected eyes became blind. We realize today that strong sunlight burns the tissue of the retina, especially the macula, since the heat rays are focused by the lens on this small area.

Under less extreme conditions the light-sensitive elements of the retina are only temporarily damaged, since the resistance of the retinal

186 KUEHN, vol. 3, p. 777. Although this sounds like a proverb, Galen obviously spoke of light sources.
187 KUEHN, vol. 3, p. 775.
188 KUEHN, vol. 3, pp. 779–780.
189 KUEHN, vol. 3, pp. 775–777.
190 SHASTID, p. 8597; KUEHN, vol. 3, p. 775 ff.

cells depends on a sufficient supply of vitamin A. Experiments demonstrated that after two months on a deficient diet the visual cells in the retina of experimental rats degenerate. By about the tenth month the animals become completely blind ... Before full destruction occurs some recovery is still possible, when vitamin A is given[191]. These experiments explain that the malnourished soldiers of XENOPHON and the prisoners of DIONYSUS had become oversensitive to the strong sunlight of the Mediterranean sky. Thus, observation seemed to support Galen's doctrine that the eye emanates a luminous pneuma which is overcome and therefore invisible in a strong illumination. However, this conclusion was evidently a logical fallacy since it was based on faulty reasoning: Galen had tried to confirm the pneumatic doctrine by observations which he explained by the very same concept which he intended to prove.

k) Definition of Color; Depth Perception by Color

Like his predecessors, especially DEMOCRITUS, PLATO and ARISTOTLE, Galen was well aware that visual impression and color sensation could not be separated. Disregarding sometimes the color effect, he spoke of light, vision and light rays *(phos, opsis, aktines)* when the physical or physiological problem was raised. This conceptual separation of color-sense from 'vision' was useful for the analysis of the problem of perception, since the color problem raised the additional question of the subjectivity or objectivity of color sensation. Even the term color involved a complex of several concepts as we will have to explain later (p. 84).

The discussion of color doctrines started in the 5th century A.D. with the three-color concept of the presocratic philosophers[192]. The interpretation of these questions became more complex in the writings of THEOPHRASTUS[193], whose treatise constitutes our main source of knowledge of these early endeavors. In a previous publication I have shown that the presocratic philosophers indicated that the various color impressions could be reproduced by mixture of three basic colors, quite similar to the modern three-color theory of YOUNG and HELM-

191 DOWLING (1966).
192 BEARE, p. 25ff. (1906).
193 STRATTON (1917).

HOLTZ[194]. PLATO and ARISTOTLE wrote in considerable detail about these questions, but their work has not yet been studied by this method[195].

Although ARISTOTLE was fully aware that many objects contained pigments, he considered these as non-essential for color perception. According to ARISTOTLE reflected light could produce a color impression even in the absence of pigment, a conclusion we can draw from his treatise *On colors*. He was, however, not explicit about the question of how the surface structure of the object produced the color, when he wrote:

> 'The bird's plumage, owing to its smoothness and the rays that fall upon it, mixed in various ways, produces various colors, just as darkness does. We do not see any of the colors as pure as they really are, but all are mixed with others, or if not mixed with any other color they are mixed with rays of light and shadows . . . All dyed things, however, take their color from what dyes them.'[196]

Although nowadays colors are produced more frequently by pigments, both natural and artificial, a great many colors result indeed from reflection of natural light from an illuminated surface which itself is colorless. We know that the many-colored tints of bird's feathers are purely the product of reflection of neutral light like the colors of the rainbow or of NEWTON's rings, since the feathers are practically free of pigment. Neither Galen nor ARISTOTLE anticipated NEWTON's explanation of diffraction of light into colors, although ARISTOTLE had already described the multicolored reflections of the rainbow[197].

Since ARISTOTLE believed that color depends on three factors: the light, the medium in space and the reflecting plane, he suggested that variations in smoothness or other qualifications of the reflecting surface could alter the color impression. To our judgement, ARISTOTLE's concept of color was basically in agreement with the atomists that a particular structure of the object of vision could create specific color

194 SIEGEL (1959). These results could be reproduced by mixing colors; watercolors present pure colors and are best suited.
195 BEARE, p. 59; ARISTOTLE, *De sensu*, 439 a 20ff.: Galen used the term *auge* for both the light of the sun and the pneumatic light-emanation of the eye, since both were not considered colored light.
196 ARISTOTLE, *On colors*, 793 b 10ff.
197 KUEHN, vol. 5, p. 640; also BOYER (1959).

sensations. Evidently ARISTOTLE recognized the importance of structure in spite of his basic rejection of the atomic doctrine.

Many apparent contradictions in the ancient doctrines of color resulted only from misunderstandings of the definition of color. The term color implies different meanings: a sensory quality resulting from the structural arrangement of the surface of the observed object; a clearly defined wave length of reflected or emitted light rays; the stimulation of a specific receptive element of the retina; and finally, a psychological phase connected with apprehending 'color'. In antiquity not all of these concepts were in use but only the first and the last.

The atomists, denying any objective existence of 'color' defined color only as a subjective sense impression of the assumed atomic structure of the object. At least, this is the commonly accepted interpretation of their teaching. ARISTOTLE and the pneumatic philosophers, however, interpreted color as an objective quality of the surface of the things seen; the transmission of the image was thought to cause simultaneous perception of form and color.

In contrast to the common belief, there is no fundamental difference between these two concepts, when we use the term color correctly, i.e., if we define the particular meaning of the term in each instance. When the atomists stated that color is a purely subjective impression (since in reality only atoms existed), they implied that our color-sensation depends upon the specific atomic structure of the surface of the object. Evidently, ARISTOTLE and the pneumatists expressed the same idea, since they considered color as the effect of an interaction between the surface of the object and the light. Color impression could only result from a specific but not necessarily atomic structure of the object's surface. Thus, both schools had a similar idea of the origin of color sensation, but used the term 'color' in a different way: the atomists for the subjective impression, the pneumatists for the condition of the surface of the object causing this color perception. We know that the early Greek philosophers were very careful about their 'definitions'. DEMOCRITUS even wrote a treatise on this subject. But this book as well as most of his other writings are lost, and since only a few scattered fragments of his treatise on color perception form the basis of modern discussion [198], the difficulties of interpretation are obvious.

Galen did not analyze the influence of color mixtures on color

198 DIELS-KRANZ, 68 b, 5 h.

perception but confined himself to a definition of color consistent with ARISTOTLE's ideas. Galen wrote that color impression resulted from the interaction between the surface of the object and the external light[199]. He defined color as 'the specific object of vision' which only the eye could perceive *(to oikeion aistheton opseos genos)*[199]. And, like ARISTOTLE, he regarded every object as a carrier of color, its color being rendered visible when its surface was illuminated by light. His concept was that color is an attribute or quality of the surface of the object. ARISTOTLE had already given an illustration of how color resulted from a transfer of qualities: thus, the 'clear air' was changed by the green color emanating from a tree with the result that all nearby objects were bathed in a green tinge[200]. Galen agreed with the idea that the green 'color' of the tree spread through the space surrounding the tree. He only substituted the term air *(aer)* for the Aristotelian term *diaphanes* (transparent medium). We find this definition not only in the writings of Galen and his contemporaries but even in modern times. A German physiologist of the last century wrote:

> 'Everything we see consists of colors spread out ... over the field of vision ... The basic constituents or elements of our visual sensation are colors.'[201]

Likewise, PTOLEMY (2nd century A.D.) stated that color was the only specific object of vision. PTOLEMY implied further that light itself was colorless (a generally accepted assumption in antiquity), since he defined color as appertaining to the surface of the object:

> 'What we see in the first line is color.'[202]
> 'Only color can be distinguished.'[203]

Galen accepted ARISTOTLE's concept:

> 'Only color but not form or size is the object of visual perception.'[204]

199 KUEHN, vol. 5, pp. 625, 639 (*anaklasis*, reflection of light) produces the colors.
200 KUEHN, vol. 5, p. 637.
201 OSTWALD (1942), quoted from LINKSZ, vol. 2, p. 52 (1952).
202 '*Illa autem que primo videtur, sunt colores*'; PTOLEMY, *Optics*, p. 13; II, chap. 5, 13.
203 '*Color solo visu dinoscitur*': PTOLEMY, *Optics*, p. 6, line 6 (pref. chap. 3).
204 KUEHN, vol. 5, p. 637, 639. This was similar to PLATO's concept (p. 26).

We also know today that changes of the intensity and quality of colors play an important role in our perception of depth. These observations were of even greater meaning to the ancients, since they did not understand the role of binocular vision for the perception of distance [205].

Galen fully supported the concept that distance could be properly judged by color perception when he wrote:

> 'Vision extends right through the air to the colored object. Recognition of size and form are based only on the color of the object. No other sense perception can perform this function with the occasional exception of tactile perception (and later: *opsei . . . hyparchei kai thesin kai diastema syndiagnoskein tou kechrousmenou somatos*).' [206]

Thus, he believed that color indicated the spatial relationship of objects at various distances. LEONARDO DA VINCI confirmed the ancient idea that space perception depended on color:

> 'There is a kind of perspective which I call aerial, because by difference in the atmosphere one is able to distinguish the various distances . . .' [207] 'Because of distance we shall lack perception of parts and outlines.' [208]

Galen was justified in relying on the concept that perception of distance depended mainly on color perception, since stereoscopic vision was not yet understood (p. 103).

4. The Role of Optics and Perspective in Galen's Doctrine of Vision

a) Introduction

During the four centuries from ARISTOTLE to Galen the studies of optics, catoptrics and perspective had made great strides. Some scientists of this period had even attempted to relate the doctrine of vision to geo-

205 See p. 101.
206 KUEHN, vol. 5, p. 625ff. (condensed). PTOLEMY made a similar statement.
207 LEONARDO DA VINCI, p. 880.
208 LEONARDO DA VINCI, p. 998.

metrical and optical laws. Well aware of this development Galen discussed these questions in two treatises dealing with visual perception: one in the tenth book of '*The function of the parts*' [209] and the other in the book of '*The commentaries on the dogmas of Hippocrates and Plato*' [210]. Although we know from his own writings that Galen was well versed in the works of the great mathematicians of antiquity such as EUCLID, HERO and PTOLEMY, we find only few references to these authors in Galen's work. The following chapter will deal first with Galen's geometrical interpretation of the visual process, then with his analysis of binocular vision. His relation to PTOLEMY and EUCLID will also be stressed.

b) Central and Oblique Rays (Figure 7)

Galen hesitated to apply the concepts of geometry or optics to his doctrine of vision because of the reluctance of his audiences to listen to such explanations. He wrote:

> 'For inasmuch as I, in connection with this matter, must touch upon the geometrical theory, an unknown subject to the majority of educated persons and one which makes them find adepts therein hated and unacceptable, I thought it preferable to omit it altogether.' [211]

With an affected modesty Galen stated that a dream had reminded him of having neglected to mention the contributions of this science to the understanding of vision and space perception. In the chapters devoted to these questions Galen employed both geometrical drawings (which have been reconstructed by modern authors) and a figurative speech to facilitate the visual comprehension of the geometrical ideas by his audience.

It has been explained previously that ARISTOTLE and the Stoic philosophers favored the concept that every type of sense perception

209 Galen, *De usu partium*, book 10; KUEHN, vol. 3, pp. 812–841. More details, see p. 48.
210 KUEHN, vol. 5, pp. 626–647; further references, see p. 48.
211 KUEHN, vol. 3, p. 812; Galen, *De usu partium*, book 10, chap. 12.

was mediated by touch, even vision (p. 174). 'Touch' by the nerves of the skin appeared as the most highly developed tactile sensation for recognition of spatial relations; smell was interpreted as 'touch' of invisible particles on the nasal surface; the same was said about liquids and air for recognition of taste and sound. The Stoics went even so far as to compare the visual emanation of the eyes to the touch of a stick in the hand of the blind. This 'stick' they stated, could be understood as a thin column of 'stretched air'.

It appears, at first, quite likely that the Stoics compared the transmission of a visual stimulus to the action of a stick in order to explain the Platonic doctrine of an assumed two-way flow of the pneuma. The 'stick' seemed to furnish a good simile, since it had first to be extended forward before a sensory impression could return along the same path to the feeling hand.

It appears, however, more convincing, that the comparison of the visual process with a stick was rather invented to convey the concept of a linear propagation of light, since the Stoics stated that during the act of vision the air between the object and the eye of the observer became tense [212] (*synentasis*, putting to a stretch). The tensile motion or vibration (*tonike kinesis*) of this part of the optically transparent medium (the area occupied by the visual axis) was thought to transmit the optical image to the eye. By speaking of a cone-shaped area of pneuma in space the Stoics had accepted a geometrical concept [213]. Like EUCLID, they postulated that the apex of the pneumatic cone was located in the eye, probably in the pupil, whereas the base touched the surface of the object of vision. In the case of a very small object only the central rays of the cone, resembling a very thin 'stick', would appear sufficient. The Stoics referred to the increased tension of pneuma in the optical cone by the term *tasis* (tension) [214]. This word was also known to indi-

212 The Stoic concept of *tasis* was different from that of the earlier philosophers. This has been discussed by Galen who was greatly influenced by the Stoics. We shall not discuss the vitalistic ideas associated with the Stoic concept of a pneuma 'extending' itself, not only through the body but throughout the entire universe as a spiritual force. We shall consider the Stoic concept of *tasis* only in relation to visual perception.

213 See CHRYSIPPUS: VON ARNIM, vol. 2, p. 233, No. 866; also see later references to ARCHIMEDES.

214 MUGLER (1957).—For reference to the Egyptian rope-stretchers (*harpenodaptai*), see DIELS-KRANZ, DEMOCRITUS No. 299.

cate both linear propagation of light or a type of linear measurement. The term *tasis* was originally a geometrical concept, a fact usually neglected in consideration of the Stoic idea of pneuma.

The term *tasis* has a long history. In ancient Egypt the early masons, carpenters and architects used a cord for measuring and laying out the ground plan of a building. A 'stretched' cord represented a perfectly straight line. Evidently, this term was also used to indicate geometrical lines. PLATO, for instance, said that the diagonal of the square is 'stretched from angle to angle'. We still call the side of a right-angled triangle opposite to the right angle *hypotenuse* (from *hypoteino*, to stretch below; the writing of the term with a 'th' is wrong; *teino* and *tasis* are derived from the same verb). The word tasis was frequently used by ARISTOTLE's commentators to indicate the visual rays because of their linear propagation [214].

Carpenters and land surveyors realized that a plumb line was shorter when fully 'stretched' between the end-points. This factor appeared important to ARCHIMEDES (born 287 B.C.), a long time before the propagation of light was fully understood. Only on a 'stretched line' could the light travel faster than on any other connection between two points. Thus, the concept of tension must have appeared of great importance for the explanation of the shortest route for the propagation of light rays. Evidently the use of the term *tasis* meant more to the Stoic scientists than an allegory, as modern readers may think: it suggested the factor of economy resulting in the rectilinear propagation of light [214].

Trying to overcome the conceptual difficulty or possibly not fully aware of the logical contradiction, the Stoic philosophers employed the concepts of *pneuma*, *tasis* and light rays often in the same context. Thus, AETIUS reported that CHRYSIPPUS spoke of the cone formed by both the optical pneuma and of fiery rays *(aktines pyrinai)* issuing from the eye. DIOGENES LAERTIUS mentioned that APOLLODORUS spoke in a similar manner of the light 'stretched in form of a cone' *(photos ekteinomenou konoeides)* [215]. But the Stoics failed to develop a consistent visual doctrine and did not apply the laws of perspective to visual problems. Nor did Galen refer to any attempt of the Stoics to reconcile the traditional pneumatic concepts with the geometrical observations and axioms.

215 VON ARNIM, vol. 2, pp. 232–234 (referring to AETIUS; ALEXANDER APHRODISIAS; DIOGENES LAERTIUS, VII, 157; APOLLODORUS).

Galen refused to compare the mechanism of vision to a stick for several reasons. He wrote that the sense of vision should not be likened to touch, since this contradicted the Aristotelian concept according to which optical impression was transmitted as a qualitative change passing through the spacefilling medium to the eye of the observer. Furthermore, he stated that a stick could communicate only the degree of hardness of an object but neither color, size nor distance. He criticized this comparison as an inference not based on facts *(syllogismos)* [216]. He also wrote that the Stoic idea of a stick had failed to explain that the visual impression *(opsis)* was reflected by mirrors at an angle of incidence [217].

However, Galen remained ambiguous when he spoke of mirror reflection, since he tried to reconcile the pneumatic with the geometrical aspect of this problem. Referring to the concept that the pneuma rebounds to the eye after having made contact with the object of vision, Galen wrote that we could speak likewise of perception by rebound along visual lines from the object to the eye. He stated that the outward-bound axial rays of the cone, after striking the object perpendicularly, had to return to the eye of the observer (*anaklasis*, the bending backwards). Galen wrote that the reflected rays (literally *gramma*, line) traveled over the same path as the outgoing rays:

> 'Therefore, the geometers can not prove it but consider it as self-evident that we see by straight lines . . . and that the angle of incidence on a mirror is the same as that of reflected light . . . If really our visual organ perceives, alone among all senses, a movement of the air as its own action, not as by a stick but as if its constituent parts had been superimposed,—provided that vision acts by reflection—then most likely a luminous pneuma streams from above to occupy the air space, and as if it would become united with itself it superimposes its [return] path on its own [path to the eye].' [218]

This idea involved certainly two assumptions: firstly, that the central rays of the visual cone were propagated rectilinearly and, secondly, that they were reflected from the object on the same path to the eye, unless we were dealing with oblique reflection from mirrors. It was an

216 KUEHN, vol. 5, p. 642.
217 KUEHN, vol. 5, p. 627.
218 KUEHN, vol. 5, pp. 626–627. ('from above' means 'from the brain'.)

essential feature for this interpretation that only the central ray could reach the optic nerve which, as Galen erroneously thought, entered the eye exactly opposite to the center of the cornea (Fig. 1). However, this geometrical doctrine did not imply a sensitization of any parts of the lens by the incoming picture as the pneumatic doctrine postulated. The oblique rays which travel at an angle to the central rays were not integrated into Galen's geometrical explanation of visual perception. Galen never mentioned that the oblique rays reach the optic nerve (at its entrance into the eyeball, opposite to the lens at the rear of the eye).

It is, however, evident to us that Galen attributed to the part of the visual field which contains the lateral, oblique rays an important role in his pneumatic doctrine of vision. Although he never referred to light rays when discussing the formation of the visual impression by the pneuma, he must necessarily have assumed that the picture *(eidolon)* was formed on the lens by the entire range of the pneumatic visual cone, since the central 'ray' could hardly produce an image larger than a point. Thus, the lateral area of the cone was needed if pneuma was to form a complete picture on the lens.

In his *geometrical* analysis of vision PTOLEMY, Galen's contemporary, had likewise failed to integrate the course of the oblique rays into the doctrine of visual perception. According to his opinion, the oblique rays neither penetrated the lens nor reached the optic nerve at its entrance in the eyeball opposite to the center of the cornea. Although PTOLEMY knew from his own experiments that obliquely incident rays are deflected in an angle at the surface between water and air, he did not speak of a deflection of the oblique rays penetrating the surface between the transparent media of the eye. He only spoke of the single central ray falling perpendicularly onto the cornea and penetrating, without deflection, to the optic nerve. PTOLEMY thus failed to apply his knowledge to the refraction of the light rays on the lens and cornea, although he defined the eye as a watery organ in contact with the outside air. Galen and PTOLEMY did not consider these already well-known optical rules of deflection as important for the problem of vision, since they could not understand that the retina accepts and transmits light rays and because they were still entirely prejudiced by the pneumatic doctrine of vision. The retina appeared merely as conductor of pneuma but not as sensory organ. Only in one respect did these authors realize the importance of oblique rays: both Galen and PTOLEMY understood that the oblique rays could cause double vision and that, therefore, perception of a single optical impression was possible only when the effect of the oblique rays was suppressed (p. 106ff.).

c) Galen and Ptolemy on Reflection

The great similarity of concepts and style suggests that the writings of PTOLEMY were a source of Galen's geometrical doctrine of vision. But it also could be an indication that the same knowledge was available to both since PTOLEMY lived simultaneously with Galen[219] (100 A.D. to 161 or 178 A.D.)[220]. Although Galen resided for many years in Alexandria where PTOLEMY lived, he never referred to PTOLEMY's scientific work.

Like Galen, PTOLEMY was convinced that vision was the result of a two-way action: of light rays leaving the eye and, after contact with the object, of rays going back to the eye. He wrote:

> 'We say that [vision] exists in two phases: one corresponding to the disposition of the object to be seen, the other to the visual act.'[221]

The assumption that the two phases of the visual act were exactly superimposed appeared as a logical basis for his geometrical treatment of optical perception and perspective. Like Galen, he spoke of the superposition of the outgoing and returning light rays (p. 90). But PTOLEMY tried to extend the idea that the light rays initially come from the eyes to the interpretation of vision by mirrors:

> 'Now it is the nature of the visual ray to proceed in a straight line from its source [in the eye] to all objects seen directly. The reflected ray, however, which proceeds from a mirror, is not in

219 It is questionable whether PTOLEMY's *Optics* was known to Galen, since PTOLEMY had composed this book rather late in life. Galen may have written his own treatise on visual doctrine some years earlier; see ILBERG (1892–1896); LEJEUNE, p. 184 (1954).

220 POLYAK (1957).

221 '*Dicimus ergo hec duobis existere modis, quorum alter fit secundum dispositionem rei videndi, alter vero secundum actum visus*', PTOLEMY, *Optics*, book 2, No. 3. *Distribuo* means 'portioning out', and therefore seems to refer to the optical or pneumatic reflection from the object to the eye. The *actus visus* denoted the process in the structures of eye.

general co-linear with the visual ray. Our senses, therefore, must have recourse to an action which is natural and customary, and so we join [mentally] the reflected ray [between object and eye] to the first part of the visual ray, the part before reflection [between eye and object]. Thus we have the impression that both parts constitute one straight ray, as it actually would be the case if nothing had happened to the ray. Hence, the image of the object will be seen as if it were an object in the direct line of sight [without an interpolated mirror].' [222]

PTOLEMY mentioned the same thought elsewhere in the following manner:

'The refracted ray coincides with the first ray, before refraction, in its position.' [223]

PTOLEMY formulated frontal vision as a modification of this idea. If a mirror image was seen at a right angle (i.e., directly in front of us), both the outgoing visual ray *(primus radius)* and the reflected ray *(fractus radius)* must travel over the same path and, therefore, the impression of a single object must appear directly in front of us [224]. Only the rays traveling to a mirror at an oblique angle do not fuse with the reflected rays [225].

In the previous chapter we quoted Galen's description of a superimposed course of both the centrifugal visual emanation and centripetal rays entering the eye. Galen's idea resembled closely the wording of PTOLEMY's treatise. This similarity could, however, be a coincidence. Evidently, both Galen and PTOLEMY described in geometrical terms an idea originally promoted by the Stoics, who had stated that the emitted and returning visual stream of pneuma traveled over the same path. Visual perception was thought to depend on this narrow 'beam' of air 'stretched' between object and eye which could be compared to a 'thin line'. Galen mentioned also the analogy between a narrow beam

222 COHEN and DRABKIN, p. 271, from PTOLEMY's *Optics*, book 3, No. 14, p. 95.
223 '*Omnia . . . coaptare que sunt de visu et lumine, ut sibi communicent, et quo ad invicem assimilatur.*' PTOLEMY, *Optics*, II, No. 1. '*Congregare radium fractium cum primo radio posito ante reverberationem.*' PTOLEMY, *Optics*, III, No. 1.
224 PTOLEMY, *Optics*, p. 95, III, No. 14.
225 PTOLEMY, *Optics*, p. 94.

of light and an almost invisible thread of a spider's web[226]. Thus, the pneumatic concept of 'stretched air' had indeed become the geometrical concept which permitted one to speak of light rays. The question, however, remained whether the pneumatic and geometrical interpretation of vision were mutually exclusive, and also whether either doctrine alone was sufficient to explain the observations. Since this philosophical problem cannot be solved by an analysis of Galen's observations and experiments, we have to discuss the general principles of his approach to the problem of vision.

d) Perception of Light Rays: A Philosophical Problem

It appeared difficult to believe that rectilinear light rays could produce a consistent picture, since they could only touch the eye at one point. But according to definition, such a point, representing the contact with a linear optical ray, could have no extension at all. EUCLID and contemporary philosophers defined a geometrical line and, likewise, the visual ray as having extension in only one dimension. It therefore appeared contradictory that points could form a plane when they had no lateral extension. But EUCLID knew that the optical image appeared extended in two dimensions and a perceptible stimulus must have spatial magnitude (p. 34).

Galen likewise thought that perception was unthinkable, if the optical image was transferred only by light rays to separate points of the sensory area of eye or brain. He searched for a solution of this logical paradox in the writings of the Greek philosophers. His answers were similar to the discussions of the Presocratics, who had already recognized the difficulties of considering a continuous line as composed of points or a plane as consistent of lines. ZENO of ELEA, formulating his answers in the form of four paradoxes, stressed also the impossibility of a logical

226 KUEHN, vol. 3, pp. 815, 817. The fact that Galen called these beams 'correlated' proves that he compared only the central 'ray' to the gossamer threads. See also the discussion of the central ray as a 'stick' of infinite thinness (p. 88). About the use of the term 'rays', see p. 90. Galen did not speak of *aktines*, the real term for rays, but of *opsis* which means visual impression. The translations from KUEHN, vol. 3, p. 815ff., refers to 'rays' (SHASTID, p. 8613; MAY, p. 493ff.; DAREMBERG, vol. 1, p. 639ff.). For Galen's use of *opsis* see KUEHN, vol. 5, p. 627. Further details, see this book p. 96.

solution if we apply geometrical ideas to physical events[227]. A comprehensive treatise on the history of philosophy, wrongly attributed to Galen, formulated similar definitions. Thus, we read:

> 'The line has no width in its length and a point has no extension in any direction.'[228]

Since Galen referred often for the study of these philosophical questions to his treatise, *On demonstration*, which has been lost[229], he did not discuss in the medical books whether a consistent picture could be formed by light rays. It follows, however, from the last quotation that he conceded that light rays must terminate at the object and the eye only in points. We also find the recognition of the logical dilemma in the contemporary writings of PTOLEMY:

> 'The visual cone has to be continuous. If it is composed of single rays then we should see points. But points are without extension and invisible, although they have a distance between themselves. Therefore, unextended points and their distances [i.e. the area not illuminated by rays] should remain invisible.'[230] [as EUCLID already discussed].
>
> 'Since points have no extension we should see nothing.'[230]

Evidently, this passage is similar to that of the pseudo-galenic treatise[228].

Although PTOLEMY did not discuss this paradox any further, it probably motivated him to state, that the visual cone was both composed of light rays and continuous in itself (a 'field' of modern terminology). On the other side, PTOLEMY postulated that reflection and diffraction are the effect only of separate light rays.

This logical dilemma was the motive that Galen preferred to assume the existence of a continuous pneumatic medium as transmitting agent of light and color. The Stoics, for the same philosophical reasons, likewise postulated pneuma as the basis of visual perception. (We may

227 SIEGEL, *The paradoxes of Zeno* (1959).
228 KUEHN, vol. 19, p. 247.
229 VON MUELLER (1897).
230 PTOLEMY, *Optics*, p. 37, book 2, No. 50.

disregard here their metaphysical and mystical motives for the assumption of *pneumata*, spirits.)

Although Galen's own pneumatic doctrine was in agreement with ARISTOTLE's concept of a continuous and undivided matter and in opposition to the atomic doctrine, Galen could not avoid speaking of light rays. In an attempt to reconcile the laws of optics and perspective with Aristotelian and pneumatic concepts Galen employed a neutral term which evidently did not contradict either doctrine and had already been employed by ARISTOTLE. The latter spoke of *opsis* as an indication of linear extension of visual emanation from the eye, and also as an expression for visual perception in the general sense. Galen adopted this terminology which evidently did not contradict his alternate doctrines of visual perception. *Opsis* meant literally 'sight', whereas the term *gamma* (line) or *aktines* (rays) had a definite geometrical overtone[231]. Thus, Galen's endeavor to account with the same expression for the pneumatic doctrine and the geometrical concept of light rays led obviously to ambiguity. He did not resolve the philosophical impasse by choosing a neutral terminology.

Furthermore, Galen realized that the finest anatomical structures could not be described as points or lines, since they were spatially extended. Fully aware of this logical necessity since he had studied in his youth geometry, mathematics and logic, Galen chose also the term *opsis* to describe the physiological and psychological aspects of vision, because this word lacked geometrical implications.

The dictionary of LIDDELL-SCOTT refers to the translation of *opsis* as 'sight, vision', but also mentions 'visual rays which were supposed to proceed from the eyes'. A review of the pertinent references supporting this translation in the dictionary showed that in the many instances *opsis* was translated as vision or sight. Therefore, the interpretative translation of *opsis* only as light rays does not appear justified. This should be considered when we consult the translations of Galen's optical treatises by DAREMBERG, MAY and SHASTID who spoke of *opsis* consistently as of light rays (rayons visuels).

In my own quotations from Galen and in the explanations in this book I tried to avoid the term light rays when Galen referred to *opsis*. The term 'sight', 'visual impression', or 'light sensation' did also imply

231 KUEHN, vol. 3, p. 818; see also footnote 226 and p. 108 for more details. ARISTOTLE, *De generatione animalium*, 781 a 4 used the term *opsis* in the double sense mentioned.

the narrow beacon of pneuma corresponding to the axial or lateral rays of the visual cone constituting the image. (See footnote 226.)

The choice of a neutral term reveals to us Galen's deep understanding of the epistemiological problem. But he could not avoid dealing in a practical way with lines and points. We know from his treatises that he supported his lectures on vision with geometrical line drawings. These have naturally been lost but were reconstructed by modern authors (DAREMBERG, KUEHN, MAY). Because these diagrams do not appear entirely consistent with the Greek text, I designed new drawings which were reproduced in this book. Special attention was given to the fact that the lateral visual lines should touch the object only tangentially (Fig. 6 on p. 104, 105). Reproductions of diagrams of the 16th century (CROMBIE, 1967) show the same errors. There is no indication that these diagrams were true replicas of the original Galenic models.

We may surmise that Galen's audience attributed to the geometrical figures the quality of being 'real', i.e. of having some form of independent existence. PLATO already wrote that it is difficult, owing to the weakness inherent in language, to distinguish the real essence of things, their understandable form, from their qualities. PLATO expressed this concept in the 7th letter to DION and in the *Timaeus*, which Galen quoted repeatedly. Likewise ARISTOTLE thought that mathematical forms existed as separate entities as W. D. ROSS remarked in his treatise on ARISTOTLE. Galen's history of philosophy (its authenticity has been doubted) pointed out that ARISTOTLE left the question open as to whether 'ideas' should be separated from matter. ARISTOTLE had indeed explained in his *Metaphysics* that there are two kinds of circles: a 'sensible' circle made of bronze or other material, and a geometrical circle which is 'intelligible' and present in the other as a 'non-sensible' substance[232]. Since Galen's interpretation of this philosophical problem was in agreement with PLATO's and ARISTOTLE's opinion, he did not consider the geometrical demonstration only as a teaching method, but as representation of reality. Modern students, however, are aware that points and lines should be regarded as abstractions.

By attributing actuality to both pneuma and geometrical concepts Galen could not escape the logical dilemma of dealing simultaneously

232 PLATO, *Timaeus*, 51 (Loeb ed.); also PLATO, *7th letter to Dion* (same vol. of the Loeb ed.) 342 E; ARISTOTLE, *Metaphysics*, 1036; ROSS, *Aristotle*, pp. 158 1959 (1956).

with two apparently contradictory doctrines of vision. To the modern scholar this problem has lost its importance. Nevertheless, the ideas of ancient science must be understood on the basis of their fundamental philosophical and epistemiological approach. Attempts of combining both doctrines into a single structure failed for a long time. I will explain in the final chapter (p. 124) that modern research was able to relate the infra-microscopical dimensions of the light-sensitive structures to geometrical points and lines. Therefore, the apparent contradictions in Galen's visual doctrine seems finally resolved (p. 126).

e) The Path of Light Rays to the Brain (Figures 3 and 4)

The geometrical analysis of visual perception rested on the concept of rectilinear light rays, since EUCLID had already proved experimentally that light rays proceed along straight lines (p. 33). Letting the light of a candle travel through a small hole of one board to an opposite board, he had demonstrated that all three points, i.e. the light of the lamp, the opening through which it passed and the light projected on the second board could be connected by a straight line[233] (p. 92). Galen wrote, without referring to these experiments: 'Visual impressions *(opseis)* are rectilinear.'[234] EUCLID's observations and writings appeared to have been Galen's main guide for the analysis of the geometrical aspects of vision.

Galen pointed out that only the central ray of the visual cone passed from the object in a straight line to the optic nerve at the rear of the eye. He had deduced from repeated anatomical studies that three points of the eye, the center of the cornea, the center of the lens and the entrance of the optic nerve into the eyeball, formed one straight line. This was, however, only approximately correct, since he overlooked that the optic nerve entered the eye slightly off-center. We know that the central ray meets the retina medially from the entrance of the optic nerve in the eye, at the 'macula', known today as the point of maximal vision (Fig. 1). Galen also failed to explain how the central ray alone could produce the picture of an object since it projected only

233 VER EECKE, p. 54.

234 DAREMBERG, vol. 1, p. 639; KUEHN, vol. 3, p. 817; Galen, *De usu partium*, book 10, chap. 12.

on one single point. In this context, Galen did not refer to EUCLID's idea that the eye had to move in order to let the axial ray travel along the object (see p. 35). But then the picture would not be formed at a single moment. Galen probably did not even consider this idea, since the necessity of such eye movements would have introduced an additional error, the time factor of motion during the visual act.

Another problem arose from the doctrine of linear propagation of light through the eyeball to the brain. Visual impressions *(opseis)* only keep their orderly arrangement corresponding to the structure of the object of vision as long as they travel through space. None of the ancient scientists mentioned how such a bundle of central rays could possibly transfer an undistorted picture through the long 'canal' of the optic nerve to the ventricles of the brain, the center of conscious visual perception (see also p. 4, 31). This difficulty remained an obstacle to the correct understanding of vision throughout the Middle Ages, until KEPLER found that the image was projected by the optical rays on the retina. But he also did not discover the correct explanation of the mode of its further transmission.

In spite of the conceptual difficulties Galen proceeded to develop a separate doctrine of vision based on the concepts of rectilinear propagation of light rays, assuming that the further course of these rays through the nervous connections between eye and brain was an equally straight path. From observation Galen wrote that the fibers of the optic nerve seemed to extend in a nearly straight line from the eye via the chiasma to the brain, where each nerve entered the lateral ventricle on the side opposite to the stimulated eye. Galen wrote:

> 'The pupil, the root of the eye, from where the nerves begin to spread [into the retina] and, thirdly, the junction of the two optic nerves entering the anterior brain lie in a straight line. They proceed on the same plane to form the eyes in the correct position that neither pupil is higher.' [235] (Fig. 3.)

Galen based his doctrine of linear propagation of the central ray through the optic nerves on the application to anatomy of one of EUCLID's propositions. EUCLID had stated that when two straight lines are

235 Galen, *De usu partium*, book 10, chap. 13; DAREMBERG, vol. 1, p. 645; KUEHN, vol. 3, pp. 830–831.

crossed, they must lie in one plane. Galen wrote that the course of the optic nerves presented two such crossing lines. Therefore, the incoming light rays must proceed on one plane from the object of vision to the brain (Fig. 4).

From the anatomical viewpoint Galen was not correct, since the axis of each eye and the optic nerves are not arranged in an exactly straight line, as could be shown by more accurate dissection or on X-rays[236]. But a superficial inspection may easily have created the wrong impression and thus explain Galen's error.

We find another contradiction in Galen's geometrical visual doctrine. When describing the function of visceral and skeletal nerves he assumed that the nervous impulse could travel along the peripheral nerves to any part of the body regardless whether or not the course of the nerve remained straight; but he did not apply this idea to the optic nerve. He disregarded completely his earlier statement that stimulation of the nerves was mediated by pneuma. The idea of a straight propagation of light through the optic nerve which contradicted Galen's pneumatic doctrine of nerve conduction was derived from misinterpretation of anatomical observations by geometrical rules.

In the 13th century ROGER BACON still wrote that 'the [image] species travelled along without refraction though caused by the power of the soul's force [i.e. pneuma] to follow the tortuosity of the nerve . . . but not along a straight line as it does in the inanimate bodies'[237].

Much later, KEPLER raised another pertinent objection to Galen's idea of a straight propagation of light rays through the optical system, stating that the movement of the eyeballs would disturb the assumed linear alignment of each eyeball with the optic nerve.

Galen thought that the optic nerves terminate at the 'thalamus' of the lateral ventricles of the brain, which he considered as the seat of conscious sense-perception (p. 4, 31). The continuation of the optic fibers from the *chiasma* to the basal ganglia of the brain and their further extension to the cerebral cortex had not yet been discovered[238]. The

236 LINKSZ (vol. 2, p. 333) wrote however only recently: 'We assume that the reason for the crossing of the optic nerves is the 'tendency' of the fibers to grow away from the eyeballs in a direction as straight as they can manage' (written in 1952). This reminds us of Galen's so-called teleology.

237 CROMBIE, *Grosseteste*, p. 155 (1953), quoting *Opus majus*, ed. Bridges, ii, 47–48.

238 Only the short part of the optic nerve between *chiasma* and *thalamus*, which is called *tractus opticus*, was known to Galen.

term *thalamus* was chosen by Galen to indicate the anterior part of the lateral ventricle from which the optic fibers seemed to arise[239]. This area of the cavity was called the 'chamber' of the optic nerve. (The Greek term *thalamus* means chamber.) In modern terminology, however, the thalamus is a large agglomeration of ganglion cells forming the medial wall of each lateral ventricle. This is another instance where a Greek anatomical term has lost its true meaning.

Galen's opinion that the optic nerves were completely crossed prevailed for many centuries. We know today that only the medial parts of the optic nerves cross. At least, this is true for the higher vertebrates and man. Only in some lower animals, especially in fish, are both optic nerves crossed completely. When we consider that in the early part of the 20th century this question had not yet been settled, it appears less astonishing that Galen was not aware of the true course of the fibers of the optic nerve[240].

f) Linear Perspective and Perception of Distance

Galen devoted more attention to the rays supposedly traveling from the eye to the object of vision than to those entering the eye from the outside. It appeared self-understood that the visual cone pointed away from the eye, its base being at the object. But the concept of the incoming rays created certain difficulties, since Galen mentioned only that the visual cone was composed of rays diverging from a point in the eye. The returning rays should, however, exhibit the same pattern, i.e. they should converge at the eye. Galen observed most certainly that the rays of a distant luminous body are divergent. But he did not apply this observation to his doctrine of vision, since he assumed that the perception relies principally on the central rays issuing from the eye toward the object.

This pattern of thought brought Galen's doctrine into conflict with the rules of linear perspective as already outlined by EUCLID who wrote that parallel lines converge toward a far point (see quotation on p. 35). We describe as the *vanishing point* the distant point of a cone, the base of which is at the eye of the observer. This is exactly the oppo-

239 Galen, *De usu partium*, book 16, chap. 3; KUEHN, vol. 4, p. 275; DAREMBERG, vol. 2, p. 164; also DUCKWORTH, p. 187. Also MAY, p. 389, n. 42; p. 687.
240 POLYAK, p. 82.

site to the visual cone of the ancients. Galen, like PTOLEMY, avoided the description of such a vanishing point, although EUCLID had already known that objects of the same size appeared smaller as their distance from the eye increased and that parallel lines meet at a distant point. Evidently, EUCLID's proposition corresponded to the ideas of modern perspective, although he described that the light rays issue from the eye in the form of a cone the base of which is at the distant object. Likewise, PTOLEMY did not formulate a correct concept of perspective, since his basic concepts were identical with those of EUCLID. However, the basic rules of perspective indicate how depth perception is perceived, even if only one eye is involved. Furthermore, the Euclidean proposition concerning the parallel lines did not depend on binocular vision. It is important to realize that the ancients treated depth perception as if it resulted from the action of a single visual organ and not from binocular vision (p. 103ff.)[241].

LEONARDO DA VINCI expressed these contrasting ideas still in the terms of antiquity:

> 'Perspective employs two opposite pyramids [i.e. cones]: one of which has its apex in the eye and its base far away at the horizon; the other has its base at the eye and its apex on the horizon. The first is embracing all the objects that pass in front of the eye; the second has to do with the peculiarity of the landscape, in showing itself so much smaller in proportion as it recedes farther from the eye.'[242]

The first idea was related to his knowledge of the ancient concept of a visual cone issuing from each eye; the second was a description of the true laws of perspective as discovered by the painters of the Renaissance.

241 EPICURUS was aware that the 'picture' or whatever is arising from the object of vision could not enter the eye in the original size of the object, but had to be gradually diminished in magnitude before entering the pupil. Later interpretation of his text suggested that the pressure of the atoms of the air on the 'picture' reduced its size during travel through space to make it fit for entering the pupil. But there is no indication that EPICURUS held this view. Obviously, the idea of a gradual diminution of a picture moving toward the eye reflects the concepts of perspective in a rather primitive form (p. 18).

242 LEONARDO DA VINCI, p. 1000 (abbreviated).—A pyramid with innumerable sides would be the approximation of a cone.

It has been mentioned before that a second type of depth perception resulted also from impression of color changes at various distances. It has no relation to the experience derived from linear perspective and the laws of geometry. It was therefore discussed in the chapter dealing with Galen's pneumatic doctrine of vision (p. 82).

g) Depth Perception, Binocular Vision and Formation of a Single Picture

Galen's and Ptolemy's Views

The first book of PTOLEMY's treatise on optics has been lost. It most likely contained a description of PTOLEMY's theory of vision. He referred briefly to the physiological problems in the other chapters, whereas the analysis of geometrical problems occupied the greater part of this treatise. In contrast to PTOLEMY, Galen dealt only briefly with the geometrical features. Therefore, the treatises of the two contemporary authors seem to furnish us with supplementary information. Some passages of Galen display even an astonishing similarity to the style and experimental details of PTOLEMY's treatise. This further supports our view that it might be permissible to reconstruct the missing features in Galen's doctrine of binocular vision from the relevant chapters of PTOLEMY's treatise. As discussed previously, it cannot be decided whether both scientists used the same sources or whether Galen was directly influenced by PTOLEMY.

Galen devoted much thought and effort to the problems of depth perception and to the question of how the simultaneous perception by both eyes resulted in the impression of a single picture. His answers were partly erroneous for two reasons: firstly, he failed to understand that psychological features played an important role in the formation of a single visual impression. Secondly, he did not recognize the great importance of binocular vision for depth perception, i.e. stereoscopic vision.

Depth Perception; The Visual Angle

Since binocular vision was not recognized as decisive for the judgement of distance, PTOLEMY explained that the idea of distance was conceived in four ways: by the apparent length of the visual rays; by the angle formed between two rays which enclose the object of vision; by the impression of the relative size of objects known to us when they stand in close proximity to the object under scrutiny; and by the changing appearance of colors according to distance (p. 82). All four types of depth perception could be performed by one eye alone. In fact, the problem of depth perception was even presented in the ancient books as a function of a single eye.

EUCLID already had postulated that an object, when seen at increasing distance, appeared to become smaller, because it was seen under a gradually diminishing visual angle. We consider this as a psychological problem, as a result of visual experience, whereas the ancients regarded it as a problem of geometry, but failed to explain how we perceive the visual angle. Since he believed in the spatial separation of the visual rays, EUCLID even thought that if a small object was moved very far away it became invisible because it would not reach from one ray to the next (p. 34); in other words it would not be touched by adjoining light rays. PTOLEMY was in full agreement with EUCLID's proposition [243], and so must have been Galen. In regard to the estimation of the length of the rays, neither PTOLEMY nor Galen explained how the eye could judge the distance of an object from the length of the visual rays presumably issuing from the eye itself.

They spoke, however, about the influence of distance on the relative size of objects as a phenomenon evidently based on experience. As mentioned before, EUCLID already referred to this factor of depth perception. Galen mentioned briefly that we hardly ever perceived an isolated object; likewise PTOLEMY discussed the rules according to which the simultaneous perception of several figures helps us to deter-

243 PTOLEMY, *Optics*, p. 37: II, No. 50; p. 19: II, No. 18.

Figure 6. Galen's description of the visual fields in monocular and binocular vision.

When looking with the right eye (R) at a column (circle) one sees the area from B over C to D; with the left eye (L) one sees the area of the column from A over B to C. With both eyes simultaneously the entire area of the column between A and D is seen. The part between B and A remains invisible to the right eye, between D and C to the left. Galen wrote that 'we see a larger area of the column with both eyes than with one eye alone' (also p. 113). He also stated that if both were used together, it appears as if the column was seen by a single eye (S) situated exactly in the middle between both eyes. (The optical lines are touching the column as tangents.)

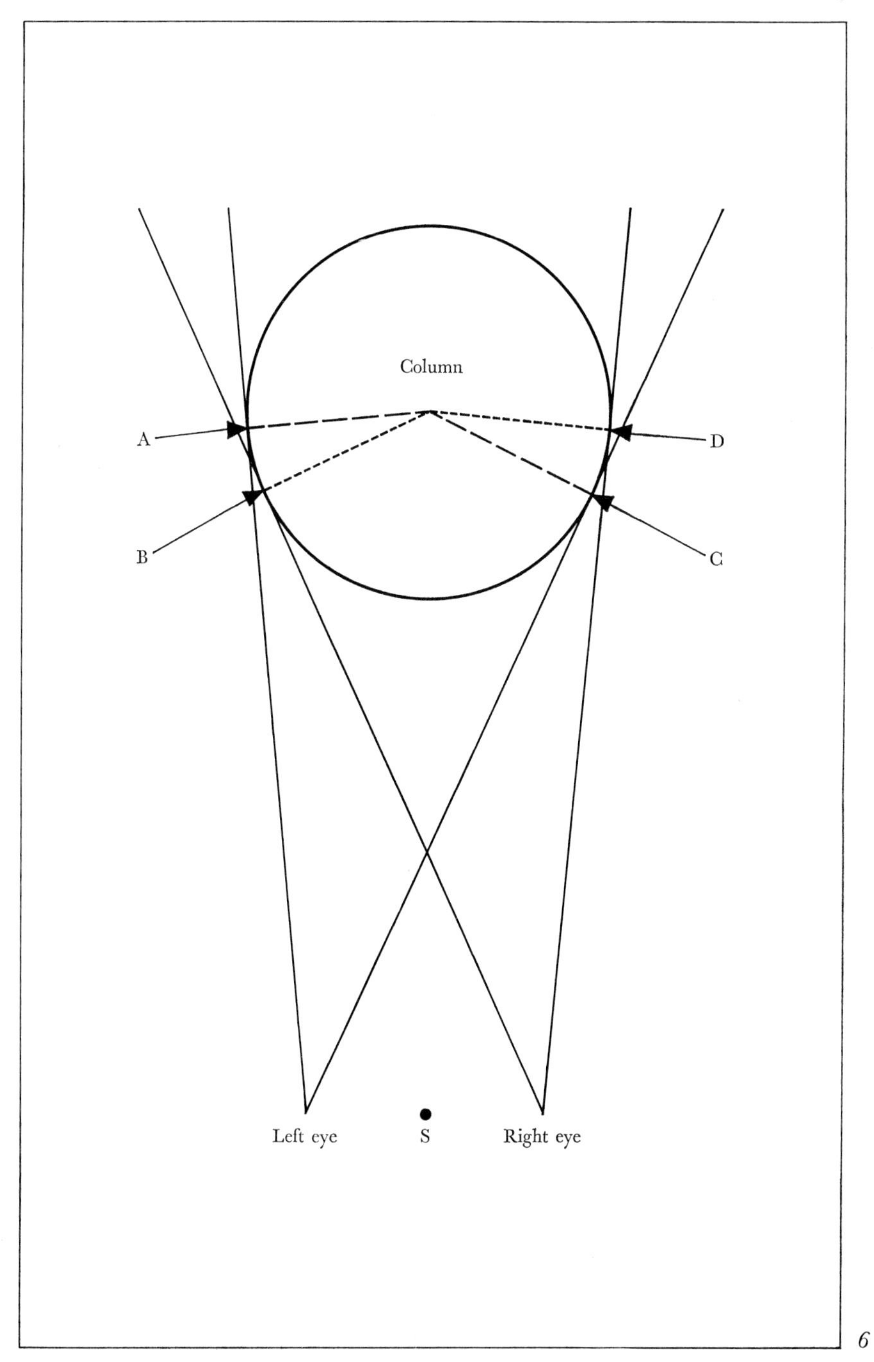
Column
A
B
D
C
Left eye
S
Right eye

mine their distance from the eye. He even attempted to measure the visual angle formed by the outlines of known objects or familiar figures as an indicator of their distance[244]. The extant writings of Galen give little information about these questions. But Galen was certainly aware that the distance of an object was judged by the images presented by the central and oblique rays[245]. Estimation of distance by color had no relation to the geometrical doctrine of vision and has already been discussed (p. 82).

Formation of a Single Picture: Diplopia and Squint

The principal question about Galen's concept of the role of binocular vision remains for us whether he also tried to explain the formation of a single picture by the coordinated use of both eyes. We know that perception of a single image by binocular vision requires only a partial overlapping of the two visual fields (Fig. 6). Man does not have the so-called 'panoramic vision' of certain animals, in which the visual fields of both eyes are contiguous without overlapping. Galen expressed this idea by stating that only the medial parts of the bases of our visual cones were superimposed, whereas we say today that the visual fields of both eyes are almost identical: i.e. they practically coincide in the vertical and horizontal plane.

Galen and PTOLEMY believed that a perfectly symmetrical alignment of both optical cones on the horizontal level guaranteed the perception of a single picture (p. 109). They did not yet know that the stimulation of corresponding points in each retina results in fusion of the two impressions into a single picture[246].

244 PTOLEMY, *Optics*, p. 49, II, No. 73. Likewise Galen, KUEHN, vol. 5, p. 639.
245 KUEHN, vol. 3, p. 817.—ROGER BACON still thought that 'magnitude was appreciated by the size of the angle at the eye . . . whence objects seen under a larger angle appear larger'. He mainly referred to ALHAZEN who, in turn, relied on Greek sources (quoted from ROGER BACON, *Opus majus*, transl. by BURKE, pt. 5, 9, 5 [vol. 2, p. 530]). BACON attributed the judgement of distance to the apparent size of several objects in the same visual field (ibid p. 524). These references illustrate the persistence of the concepts of the Hellenistic and therefore the galenic optical doctrine. EUCLID's description of the relation between the visual angle and the apparent size of the object is illustrated by a drawing of 1703, reproduced by CROMBIE, p. 8 (1967).
246 We know today that only stimulation of corresponding points of both retinae produces a single picture. ARISTOTLE's remark concerning the formation of a single picture by stimulation of corresponding points in the 'eyes' referred probably to the lens, but not to the retina (p. 32). It was not mentioned by Galen.

Galen explicitly stated that, in order to perceive a single picture, the basis of each visual cone must rest at the surface of the object. In describing this mechanism he defined the visual impression *(opseis)* surrounding the axial area of the cone (the gray area in Fig. 7) as 'correlated', since it was directed toward the center of the object of vision. The peripheral area of the cone he called uncorrelated impression *(opseis)*. He wrote:

> 'All those visual impressions *(opseis)* which stand at equal intervals from the axis and reach the same given plane [i.e. the base of the cone resting on the object], we will call correlated visual rays (*homotageis*, literally: equally arranged); the other lines [i.e. rays] however, we call uncorrelated.'[247]

Thus, the position of the eyes was indicated by the pathway of the correlated, i.e. central rays of the cone.

Galen recognized that visual fusion of the two optical impressions was mediated by a postural factor resulting from a coordinated action of the eyes, since he observed that an object, when seen by each eye alone, appeared at a different position (see Fig. 7). He wrote:

> 'An object, when seen with both eyes, always appears to stand in a different place from that where it seemed to be when gazed upon by either eye.'[248]

He explained further that an object when seen with both eyes 'appears in a third position', i.e. in the middle between the two spots where the separate impressions of each eye were observed.

Galen was, however, convinced that the fusion of the two optical impressions depended merely on a perfect adjustment of both eyes in the horizontal level. But he indicated that only the position of the axial rays was important, since these alone were supposed to reach the optic nerve:

> 'The axis of the visual cones must be in one and the same plane, in order that what is single may not appear double . . . The optical

247 KUEHN, vol. 3, p. 817; SHASTID, p. 8613.
248 SHASTID, p. 8614; KUEHN, vol. 3, p. 821.

canals [i.e. both optic nerves] must also be constructed on one and the same plane.'[249]

The exact positioning of the eyes in the horizontal plane seemed to prevent double vision, even when the optical axes (central rays) were not accurately centered on the same point of the object. Galen made the erroneous statement that even in a case of horizontal squint the light rays could still travel in a straight line from the object through each eye toward the sensory center of the opposite brain (see p. 99 and KEPLER's critique of this doctrine p. 100)[250].

PTOLEMY described the coordination of both eyes on one plane in terms similar to those of Galen, likewise referring only to the central rays.

249 KUEHN, vol. 3, p. 828ff.; SHASTID, p. 8617; Galen, *De usu partium*, book 10, chap. 13; PTOLEMY, *Optics*, p. 27, II, No. 28. This sentence agrees with the previous unchanged text of Galen. The emendation of KUEHN, vol. 3, p. 825 as proposed by MAY (p. 497, footnote 62) does not change the meaning.
250 CROMBIE, *Kepler*, op. cit.

Figure 7. Galen's concept of single and double vision (lateral and central rays).

Part I. If the observer looks at the white column (light circle) with the left eye (L), the black column (dark circle) appears momentarily to the left of the black column; if the white column is fixed by the right eye (R), the black column will appear momentarily to the right of the white column. These momentary impressions are represented in the drawing by a dark half-circle (A and B). The visual cone of the left eye is indicated by the entire shaded area. The dark central lines correspond to the central (axial) rays of the visual cone which transmit the impression of the column. The lighter (outer) shaded area of the visual cone indicates the field of the oblique rays. The oblique rays terminate on the lens, whereas the axial (central) rays, pass through the lens and reach the optic nerve at its entrance into the eyeball (at the optic disc).

Part II. If the observer looks at the white column suddenly with both eyes, a double image of the black column becames visible for a short moment. This fleeting double image remains unsharp, since the black column is not in the path of the axial (coordinated) rays. Indeed, the double image will quickly disappear when we concentrate only on the sharp (central) picture of the column. In the drawing (II) the double images are indicated by the half-circles.
Note that Galen did not only speak of rays but of *opsis*, of visual impression as explained in detail on p. 94, 96.

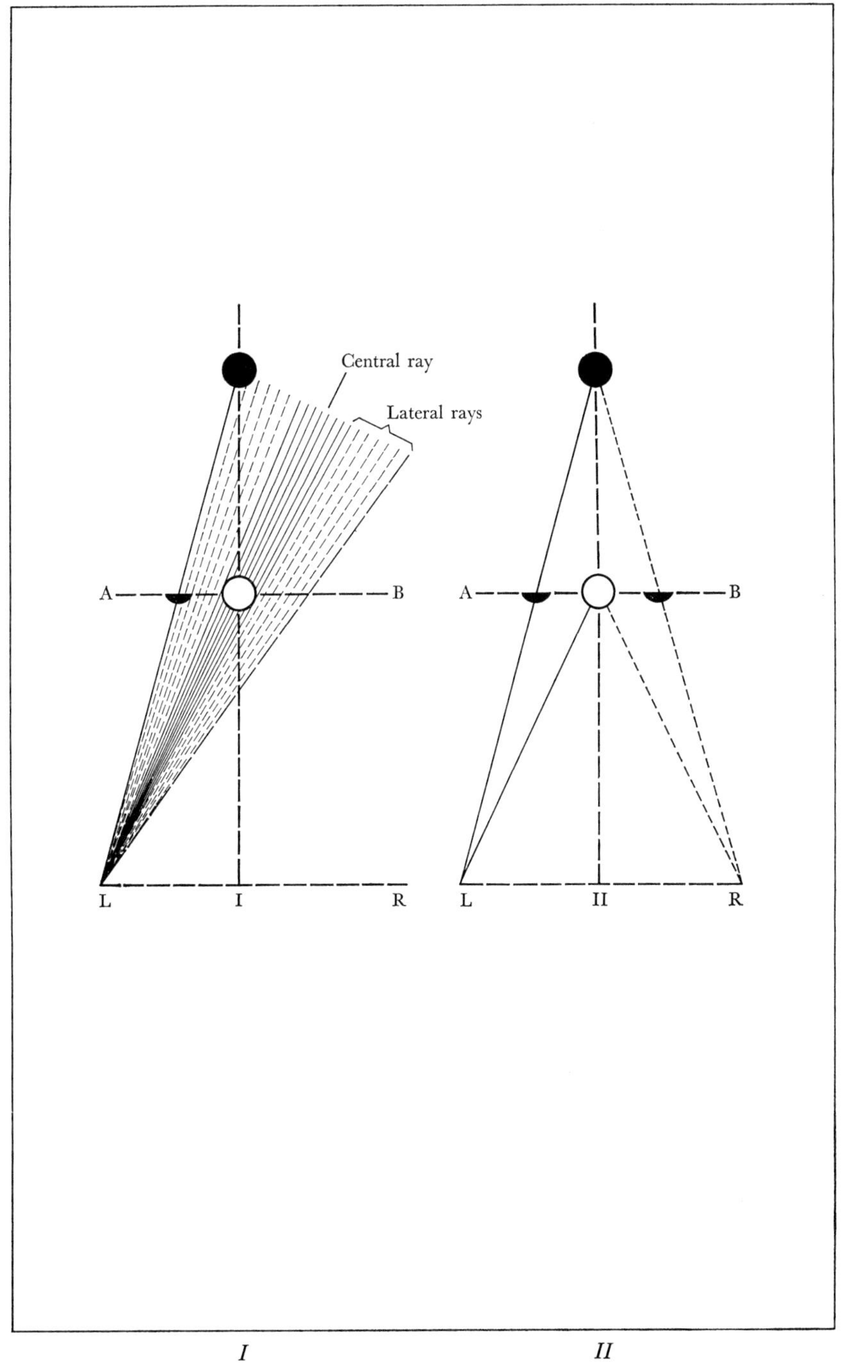

I *II*

7

'An object appears in one place and on the same plane when seen with one eye [i.e. laterally if compared to the position where it would be, if seen by the other eye]. But when seen with both eyes it is perceived in another place [i.e. between the places to which each eye alone would project it, but at the same level plane], because it is seen with correlated rays *(radiis consimilibus)* which occupy the same position in each pyramid [251] [i.e. cone] in relation to the axis of each.' [252] (see Fig. 6).

PTOLEMY explained this further:

'Obviously nature created vision with both eyes that we can perceive more, and also more orderly and conclusively . . . Both [optical] axes should fall on the middle of the object of vision so that the bases of both visual pyramids [251] are united at the contact with the object.' [253]

PTOLEMY even attempted to prove experimentally that fusion was guaranteed, when both pyramids remained on the same horizontal plane as both optic nerves and the chiasma: he temporarily produced double vision by pressure on the eyeball from below or above.

Galen described a similar experiment: when he pressed one eye upward or downward, the visual axis of this eye was displaced from the common plane on which both eyes had been before. Therefore, horizontal fusion of both visual images became impossible. Galen distinguished this type of double vision from the common (horizontal) squint in which one eye is deviated laterally. Galen explained the diplopia by vertical shift according to a proposition from the 11th book of the *Elements* of EUCLID, from which he deduced that the optical rays could not fuse when they were displaced from the horizontal plane on which both eyes and the optical nerves were normally located (p. 107, Fig. 3, 4).

251 Pyramid or cone had the same meaning; a pyramid with an infinite number of sides at the base would be a cone.
252 PTOLEMY, *Optics*, p. 26, book 2, No. 27.
253 PTOLEMY, *Optics*, p. 27, II, No. 28. This described indeed the overlapping of both visual fields according to modern terminology.

'When two straight lines intersect they lie in one single plane, since every triangle is placed on one single plane.' [254]

This argument does not impress us as convincing. We know that Galen drew wrong conclusions from dissections and also that horizontal (lateral) squint was—and still is—the most commonly encountered displacement of the eyeballs, but that it rarely causes double vision. The reasons for the suppression of a second image are purely psychological and better understood today than at Galen's time. When the squinting eye receives an optical impression the mind suppresses its conscious perception. The result is that, after a long time, the deviated eye becomes blind or at least very weak. Since Galen was not aware of this fact, he thought that fusion necessarily occurs in horizontal squint. Vertical deviation of one eye, however, seemed in most instances, to result in diplopia. But Galen had failed to recognize the importance of the time factor for adaptation to squint, since he produced the vertical deviation of the eye by a sudden pressure on the eyeball.

Evidently, in Galen's experiment with vertical deviation of one eye, the time was too short for the adaptation, i.e. for learning to suppress the second image. More careful evaluation of his observations should have suggested to Galen that the short duration of this experiment did not permit the patient to overcome the sudden disturbance by an unconscious mental process. Galen also failed to recognize that lateral pressure on the eyeball could cause momentary diplopia. He further overlooked that in permanent squint the second picture was mentally eliminated, and that ultimately the deviated eye ceased to function [255]. He was guided only by the observation of the end-result of congenital (lateral) squint, but was not motivated by psychological considerations, when he wrote:

'It is not every distortion [of the position] of the pupil which makes an object appear double, but only the shift which carries the pupil upward or downward from its natural position. The displacement toward the larger or the smaller canthus [i.e. the external or internal angle of the eye] only causes the object to appear more to the

254 KUEHN, vol. 3, p. 830 (Galen referred to the 11th book of EUCLID's *Elements*).
255 LINKSZ, vol. 2, p. 556. The optical nerves form indeed two triangles at the chiasma (see fig. 3) which almost are on the one level.

left or to the right, but certainly not double, since the axes of the visual cones remain in the same plane . . . and neither of the pupils stands higher.'[256]

In his treatise on optics, PTOLEMY hinted that binocular fusion on the horizontal plane could be the result of psychological adaptation[257]. But Galen tried to relate fusion of the two optical impressions to his pneumatic doctrine, assuming that the two separate incoming pictures were combined into one when the streams of pneuma from each eye unite at the chiasma, the crossing of the optical 'canals' (nerves)[258]. He wrote:

'The purpose of the junction of the nerves is the prevention of double vision.'[259]

We notice here again Galen's lack of a clear distinction between geometrical and pneumatic ideas.

Earlier in this chapter, it was discussed that Galen explained depth perception by monocular vision. His writings did not give any indication that he ever attributed the perception of depth to stereoscopic (binocular) vision, since he thought that two different visual impressions arriving in the brain would lead to diplopia. The next chapter will discuss his concept of the purpose and advantage of binocular vision.

Purpose of Binocular Vision

The question still remains unanswered as to what purpose Galen attributed to binocular vision. Observation seemed only to suggest that

256 KUEHN, vol. 3, p. 826.
257 LEJEUNE, p. 146 (1948).
258 KUEHN, vol. 3, p. 814 and pp. 836–837.
259 KUEHN, vol. 3, p. 836.—ROGER BACON (1214–1292) referred to the same observation and almost with the same words. 'But it is necessary that the two *species* coming from the eyes should meet at one place in the common nerve . . . and become one form . . . A proof of this is the fact that when the species do not come from the two eyes to one place in the common nerve, one object is seen as two. This is evident when the natural position of the eyes is changed, as happens if the finger is placed below one of the eyes or if the eye is twisted somewhat from its place; both species do not then come to one place in the common nerve, and one object is seen as two' (quoted from ROGER BACON, *Opus majus* v.i.v. 2, ed. Bridges, ii. 32–33, by CROMBIE, *Grosseteste*, p. 154 (1953).

binocular vision offered the advantage of a slightly wider visual field (Fig. 6). EUCLID had written:

> 'If one looks at a cylinder [or a column] with one eye, one sees less than a demicylinder . . . but with both eyes one sees the entire half of the cylinder.' [260]

We know that Galen was familiar with EUCLID's work; but it is also possible that he found this idea in PTOLEMY's treatise. Galen noticed that binocular vision seemed evidently to grant not only a wider view of the object than a single eye but also revealed the relation to surrounding objects. Galen wrote:

> 'An object hides less [of itself] when seen with both eyes than when seen with one eye only.' [261]

Galen wrote further that we also see a wider area with both eyes than with one eye alone:

> 'Every object which is to be perceived is never seen isolated by itself, but always something is seen by the visual rays which pass around it and which proceed, at times, to an object on the hither side of the thing which is looked at; at times, however, to some object on the thither side.' [262]

Thus the advantage of binocular vision was to open the view to a larger field and to reveal objects often not seen by one eye alone.

Galen's observations were correct: when we stand near a column and close first one and then the other eye, we will find that certain lateral parts of the column appear only to one eye: with the right we see a section of the right side of the column which remained invisible to the left eye, and vice versa [263] (Fig. 7).

It is of interest that PTOLEMY described the same experiment but came to conclusions different from and more far-reaching than those of Galen. When Galen referred to the lateral shift of each column, he did

260 VER EECKE, p. 20.
261 KUEHN, vol. 3, p. 823.
262 SHASTID, p. 8613; KUEHN, vol. 3, p. 818. See also KUEHN, vol. 5, p. 639.
263 KUEHN, vol. 3, p. 822; SHASTID, p. 8615.

not mention that the surrounding objects appear unsharp. PTOLEMY, however, directed his attention equally to the surrounding objects. In the experiment with two columns, one white, one black, PTOLEMY found that one column appeared indeed double when the eye was fixed upon the other. PTOLEMY proved the reason for this shift by a strictly geometrical analysis. He showed that the column which was not in the path of the central rays had to appear double because it remained outside the path of the central (coordinated) rays, and therefore was not in the line of the two visual axes (Fig. 7). Everybody who repeats this simple experiment will obtain the same result as PTOLEMY.

PTOLEMY recognized that the oblique (uncoordinated) rays form only an indistinct visual impression, but he did not state specifically that we are usually not aware of double pictures in the peripheral field. He noticed the same phenomenon on mirrors, where oblique rays seemed to produce a less distinct picture than the axial rays [264].

Evidently, the only difference between Galen's and PTOLEMY's analysis of these observations was that Galen failed to refer to the double picture formed by the second column. He also did not even mention that the peripheral vision appeared unclear when he had focused his eyes on the first column.

Today we understand the experiment with the columns better, since we realize that the suppression of the second image of the column is a psychological act. It takes, however, great concentration during these experiments to become aware of the double image as anyone can easily convince himself.

In conclusion, Galen thought that binocular vision was advantageous because it opened a larger field of vision, but PTOLEMY recognized also disadvantages of the larger field, their unsharp outlines and

264 LEJEUNE, p. 185 (1958); PTOLEMY, *Optics*, p. 19.

Figure 8. Medieval concept of the central rays entering the optic nerve.

This simplified diagram is designed after an elaborate drawing in an Arabic manuscript of the 15th century [1]. Its author followed Galen's concept that only the central rays enter the optic nerve, whereas the oblique rays do not penetrate beyond the lens.

1 For details about the Arabic drawing, see POLYAK, fig. 348, p. 556 (1957).

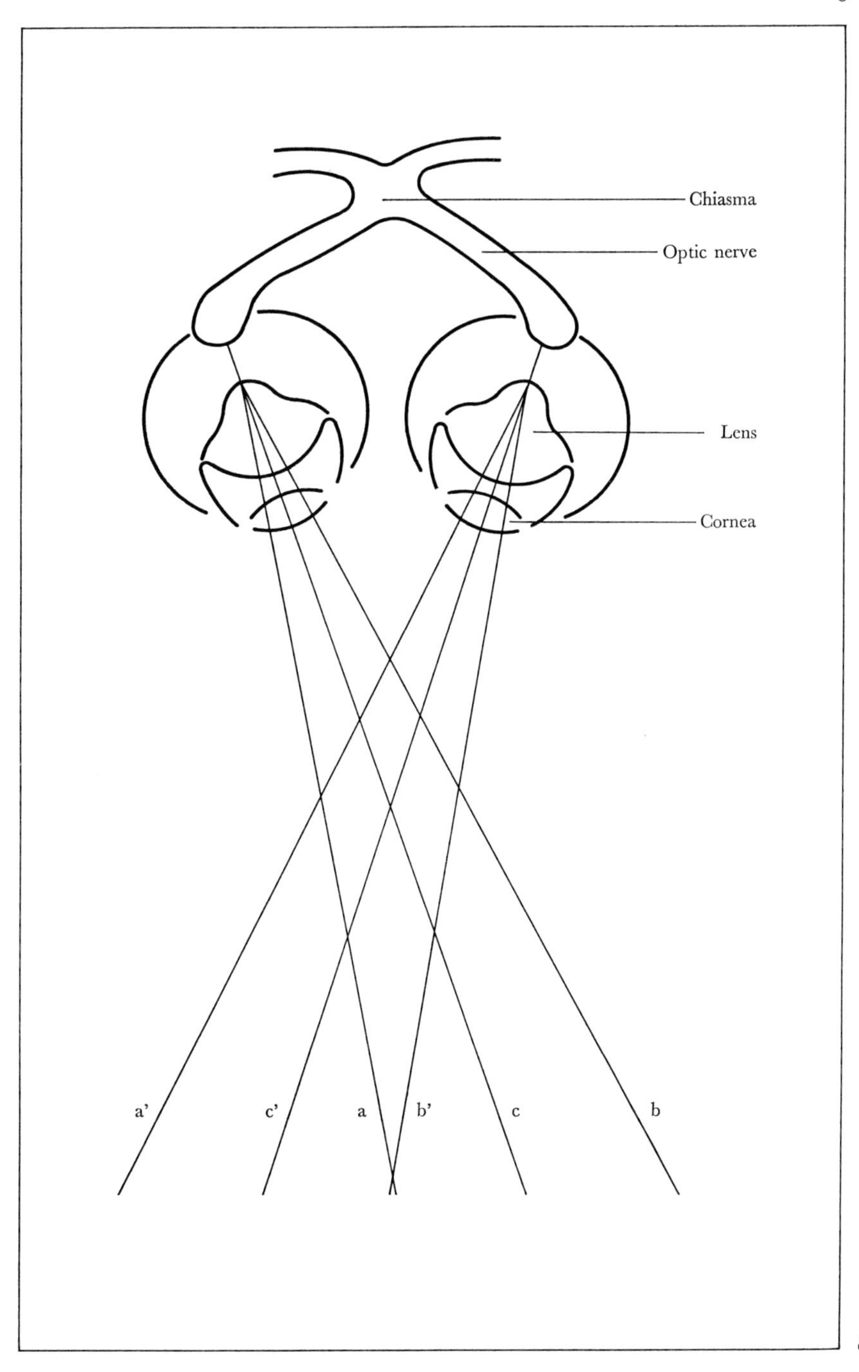
Chiasma
Optic nerve
Lens
Cornea
a'
c'
a
b'
c
b

the double-images in the peripheral areas. But both failed to understand that stereoscopic vision facilitated depth-perception.

For a long time the studies of the role of axial or central rays for visual perception remained under the influence of Galen's and PTOLEMY's teaching. The famous Arabic physician ALHAZEN (p. 12) ignored the oblique rays entirely, but overemphasized the role of the perpendicular (central) rays (Fig. 8). He refuted, however, the doctrine that a visual emanation issued from the eyes. He still believed that the image was formed either in the lens or in the vitreous. But his text remained ambiguous about the exact location of the image. He certainly did not believe that the incoming rays stimulated the retina, whereas he assumed that the light rays passed through both the central and lateral areas of the lens into the optic nerve [265].

Galen's erroneous concept that the rays travel rectilinearly to the optic nerve was maintained until refraction by lenses became understood shortly before 1300 [266]. Still in 1589, GIAMBATTISTA DELLA PORTA was teaching that a visual image was formed at the surface of the lens. This reminds us that Galen had compared the lenticular capsule to a mirror (p. 52). Then, FELIX PLATTER discovered in 1583 that the retina is the true photoreceptor [267]. KEPLER made it finally clear (1603) that all optical rays, including the oblique ('collateral') rays, were refracted by the lens. He also discovered that all rays form a picture on the retina, but stated that the picture of the direct rays is clear, whereas that induced by oblique rays remains unsharp as PTOLEMY had explained. He also was not yet consistent about the refraction by lens and cornea, since his text and diagram were contradictory. He formulated his discovery of refraction still in the terminology of the ancients when he wrote in the treatise *Ad Vitellionem paralipomena:*

> 'The axis of the direct cone is not refracted at the cornea, whereas the axes of the oblique ones are refracted there.' [268]

Although KEPLER described the refraction of the light rays by the eye in great detail, he still retained Galen's pneumatic doctrine of nerve

265 Figure 8 is a diagram made after a photograph from a medieval manuscript reproduced by POLYAK (1957).
266 POLYAK, pp. 19, 29, 35, 39, 85; MEYERHOF (1920).
267 POLYAK (1957).
268 CROMBIE, *Kepler*, p. 157.

conduction of the visual stimulus and tried to reconcile this doctrine with his own optical discoveries:

> 'The sensory power or spirit, diffused through the nerve, is more concentrated and stronger where the retina meets direct [optical] cones, because of its source and where it has to go ... For this reason oblique vision satisfies the soul least.'[269]

The fallacy of assuming an active pneuma in the lens was ultimately demonstrated by FELIX PLATTER when he cut the fibers connecting lens and retina (even the *zonula Zinnii*; p. 57). This ingenious experiment proved that vision was still possible when the lens had been detached from all connection with the retina. This was the first experimental proof that the interior structures of the eye were purely optical instruments[270]. PLATTER, however had not disproved that pneuma passed through the optic nerve to the retina.

It was the purpose of the preceding chapters to explain Galen's mode of thinking. His conclusions were derived from concepts prevailing at his own time. They appear understandable only when seen against the background of *Hellenistic* science and philosophy. Galen's doctrine of vision became obsolete after it had served its purpose, but not until new discoveries and philosophical concepts had given fresh impulse to biological science.

E. DECLINE OF SCIENTIFIC METHOD AFTER GALEN: PLOTINUS ON THE DOCTRINE OF VISION

Hellenistic science did not produce another doctrine of vision comparable to that of Galen. The few ophthalmological treatises of late antiquity which have been preserved deal mainly with diagnosis and therapy of eye diseases. A detailed discussion of visual problems can, however, be found in the philosophical treatise of PLOTINUS (203–270 A.D.). Born in Egypt, he lived in Alexandria before he emigrated to Rome in the year 244. He is known as the founder of the Neoplatonic School of philosophy, and he was much devoted to mysticism, even in

269 CROMBIE, *Kepler*, pp. 157–158.
270 POLYAK, p. 35.

his discussion of the problems of vision. Thus, he wrote that the soul, spreading out through the universe, had eventually to come to rest, like light which only could shine for a limited time before turning into darkness [271].

PLOTINUS' discussion on visual perception raised the question of Galen's influence on the writers of the Hellenistic time period. In contrast to Galen, PLOTINUS' approach to the problems of visual perception remained deductive, since he failed to support his views by observation and experimentation. Although his familiarity with the work of the preceding writers is evident, he did not quote the earlier authors, not even PTOLEMY or Galen.

PLOTINUS' discussion of vision illustrates the decline of medical science which started soon after Galen's death. PLOTINUS presented his doctrine of vision in a poorly arranged manner, since ill health forced him to ask his pupil PORPHYRY to edit his handwritten but uncorrected notes. PORPHYRY's book bears the title *On the life of Plotinus and the arrangement of his works* [272]. His edition of the 5th chapter of the 4th *Ennead* of PLOTINUS contained a section which bears the title *Problems of the soul, or on sight.*

In this chapter PLOTINUS discussed most of the traditional explanations of the visual process. Thus, without referring to EPICURUS or any other member of the atomistic school, PLOTINUS declared that the image *(eidolon)* of an object of vision would have to divide the air during its course to the eye, but that the resistance of the air would retard its progress [273]. The fact that an object was visible from many sides and in all parts of the space, regardless of the position of the observer, seemed to render the idea of a traveling picture *(eidolon)* unacceptable [274]. On the other hand, PLOTINUS could not conceive that a picture traveled through empty space.

Many scientists of antiquity had considered air as the most likely medium of optic transmission. PLOTINUS, however, regarded it as impossible that air could conduct the visual impression. He based his objection on the idea that we observe other worlds, separated from our own cosmos by a distance, vast and void of air. Therefore, PLOTINUS reasoned, our vision could hardly depend on a medium consisting prin-

271 PLOTINUS, *Enneades*, IV, 3, 9.
272 MACKENNA (1932, reprinted 1966).
273 PLOTINUS, *Enneades*, IV, 5, 2.
274 PLOTINUS, *Enneades*, IV, 5, 2 and 3.

cipally of air [275]. Furthermore, he believed that there was a fundamental difference between the transmission of light and heat, the latter definitely requiring the air for its transport [276]. This left him with no alternative but to propose that light itself filled the space (*metaxy*, literally, in between).

PLOTINUS did not discuss the traditional question of whether light was transmitted as a continuous space-occupying agent or by rectilinear rays. Merely speaking of 'light' as such PLOTINUS referred to its two sources: the eye, and the object itself.

PLOTINUS opposed the doctrine of light as an emanation issuing from the eye, for reasons similar to those discussed in an earlier chapter: an observer would have to be aware of the object before he could even perceive it; he even would have to know its location before he directed his gaze upon it (p. 71). This would require an act of memory *(mneme)* which appeared obviously impossible [277]. PLOTINUS further objected that, according to the doctrine of visual emanation, a beam of light had to be extended from the eye like a 'stick' in order to find its object; further, the object needed to offer resistance, since the rebound of the emanation had to be communicated to the eye. This concept appeared to him similar to the idea of a medium in space, which he had already refuted as a logical impossibility [277].

This impasse seemed to leave no other alternative than simply to speak of light coming from the object of vision. But at this point PLOTINUS' ideas became more involved and even contradictory. He reasoned that, since space was dark and darkness was a material entity [278], an external illumination of the object was definitely required. This, he thought, could only apply to distant *(porro)* objects. But if the object of vision was close-by it should be visible without illumination from the outside. PLOTINUS stated indeed that the light of another source *(allotriou)* was not required for 'simple vision' *(haplos horan)* of nearby objects [279]. He failed, however, to ascertain whether the light needed for close vision originated in the eye or in the object itself. We can only surmise from PLOTINUS' extensive discussion of the so-called 'sympathetic contact' that he was thinking of an initial sympathetic transfer

275 PLOTINUS, *Enneades*, IV, 5, 3 and 6.
276 PLOTINUS, *Enneades*, IV, 5, 2 and 4.
277 PLOTINUS, *Enneades*, IV, 5, 4.
278 PLOTINUS, *Enneades*, IV, 5, 2.
279 PLOTINUS, *Enneades*, IV, 5, 4.

of light from the eye to the object of vision. The term 'sympathy' was a physiological concept in Galen's system of medicine, but a psychological idea for PLOTINUS who related it to the concept of soul.

We will come to a clearer understanding of the predicament in PLOTINUS after a discussion of the concept of qualities which he understood in obvious analogy to Galenic ideas. We shall ultimately recognize that PLOTINUS neither accepted the interpretation of the propagation of light as an extension of qualities between object and eye nor that he was satisfied with a sympathetic doctrine of light which seemed likewise to involve logical contradictions.

Evidently in agreement with his denial of a space-filling corporeal agent, PLOTINUS discussed the idea that qualitative changes of an undefined intermediary agent (*metaxy*, in between, an adverb used as noun) could transmit the visual impression to the observer. Unable to specify the nature of this medium, he likened it to the rod and line of the harpoon through which the paralyzing shock of the electric torpedo-fish was transmitted to the fishermen [280]. The harpoon, however, did not undergo any visible changes when it conveyed the often lethal stimulus to the harpoonist (PLOTINUS called the transmitted stimulus *pathos*, affection) [281].

Galen already had been greatly impressed by the observation of this powerful yet unknown quality *(poiotes)* issuing from the torpedo-fish. In fact, the communication of a paralyzing effect by the torpedo-fish furnished Galen with an important argument in support of the doctrine of pneumatic transmission which he also applied to the explanation of the transfer of the visual image. Galen proposed on the basis of these considerations that an unknown quality of the pneuma was conducted through the space, similar to the specific dynamis or quality which was the assumed mediator of the stimulus along the nerves. PLOTINUS, however, did not discuss this important doctrine in detail nor did he refer to Galen's doctrine.

Like Galen, PLOTINUS presumed, however, that light perception was based on a quality of the object [282] and could thus be considered as a form of energy *(energeia)*, as an active force which other authors defined as *dynamis* [283]. Since PLOTINUS thought that such a force emanat-

280 SIEGEL, pp. 149, 177, 360–382 (sympathy) (1968); see also this book p. 72 ff.
281 PLOTINUS, *Enneades*, IV, 5, 1.
282 PLOTINUS, *Enneades*, IV, 5, 6.
283 SIEGEL, p. 183 (1968).

ing from the object of vision did not require another medium *(metaxy)* for transmission [284], he identified light with energy. This idea contradicted Galen's concept of light as the activity of the *cerebral* pneuma.

In earlier chapters we mentioned that Galen had failed to separate strictly the terms *pneuma*, *dynamis* (force) and quality *(poiotes)*, and that the use of these terms as synonyma made Galen's physiological doctrine difficult to understand. According to PLOTINUS, light as an immaterial energy needed only space, since it arrived at the eye by extending itself through the void. PLOTINUS wrote:

'Light is the energy of a luminous body directed outward.' [285]

PLOTINUS concluded that the light itself should be regarded as incorporeal. Likewise he did not consider the energy of sunlight as a material emanation. Color seemed to be identical with light, since only the surface of light-emitting bodies appeared colored [285]. This was a repetition of the Aristotelian idea, which Galen also had accepted. But PLOTINUS never mentioned Galen, possibly because the latter did not define the qualities as immaterial even though they were weightless.

In spite of many similarities to Galen's doctrine, PLOTINUS had practically refuted all preceding concepts of vision, even ARISTOTLE's idea of the *diaphanes*, the hypothetical, stationary, transparent medium of vision. However, PLOTINUS' idea that light itself was its own transmitting agent was a tautology, since it indicated only that light is visible. When PLOTINUS spoke of light as a radiating energy, he even drifted into mystic speculations. His comparison of the energy of light to the soul proved undoubtedly the influence of the Stoic concept of pneuma. But we should remember that the Stoics had a materialistic concept of the pneuma [286] whereas PLOTINUS spoke of light as incorporeal.

PLOTINUS mentioned that there was no need to consider light as a separate agent, since the *psyche*, the soul, could account for the visual contact *(haphe)* over the distance *(diastema)* separating the object from the observer [287]. This hypothetical function of the immaterial soul suggested to PLOTINUS the already mentioned idea of '*sympathy*' as the basis of visual perception.

284 PLOTINUS, *Enneades*, IV, 5, 6 and 7.
285 PLOTINUS, *Enneades*, IV, 5, 7.
286 SIEGEL, pp. 143, 146 (1968).
287 PLOTINUS, *Enneades*, IV, 5, 4.

The concept of sympathy was discussed in my previous book in relation to Galen's physiological doctrine [288]. Galen described different types of sympathy (i.e. correspondence). He thought that an irritant could simultaneously render several organs diseased, or that an irritant such as black bile, secreted by spleen or stomach, could affect (by sympathy) in successive stages distant parts of the body. Galen remained contradictory about the physical mode of sympathetic transmission of disease by such hypothetical agents through the body. In other instances, Galen related the transmission of sympathy to the neural connection between distant organs, as i.e. by vagus fibers between stomach and brain. Galen always considered sympathy as a process of material nature. He never took recourse to mystic forces and avoided speaking of an immaterial soul. He stated that even if the soul existed we would never be able to understand it [289].

Similar considerations hardly disturbed PLOTINUS. The idea that the soul occupied fully the 'void' between eye and object seemed to eliminate the necessity of searching for a corporeal visual medium. It also seemed to eliminate the controversial concept of an empty space. On the other hand, PLOTINUS expressed great doubts about the validity of this argument. He reasoned that only if we postulate a functional sympathetic unity of all three components, the eye, the space and the object of vision, can we consider the soul as responsible for visual perception. It appeared, however, unlikely that soul or body, as physical units, were able to perceive the parts which constitute a whole. Further, if the visual organ would be able only to perceive objects sharing similar qualities, then it could not become aware of the presence of outside objects composed of qualities alien to it. Thus, PLOTINUS reasoned that the living organism could recognize neither the cognate parts of itself nor external objects of dissimilar composition. PLOTINUS, therefore, came to the conclusion that the soul could not be the visual medium nor sympathy could really mediate the visual process. Even the philosophical concept of sympathy appeared to him as an unsuitable answer to the problems of vision [290].

As it seems, we are left without any concise idea of PLOTINUS' doctrine of vision, if he had formulated such a doctrine at all, since sophistic reasoning had led him into an impasse similar to the discussion of

288 SIEGEL, pp. 360–382 (1968).
289 SIEGEL, pp. 108, 192 (1968).
290 PLOTINUS, *Enneades*, IV, 5, 8.

the four paradoxes by ZENO [291]. This mode of thought was, however, entirely alien to Galen who would never have accepted the idea of space and body as a living unit imbued by 'soul'. Galen even did not want to discuss the problem of the nature of the soul.

PLOTINUS also touched briefly the problems of visual perspective, again without mentioning the earlier geometrical treatises dealing with these questions. We find in the *Enneades* a short chapter bearing the title *Why distant objects appear small* [292]. Without referring to other sources, PLOTINUS wrote that we could judge distance by comparing the relative size of objects known to us. He even referred to color perspective, stating that distant colors appeared dim [293]. He also denied that the visual angle could be a useful measure of distance, since the impression of a large mountain or of the whole sky occupied the entire field of vision, even if they were far removed from the observer [294]. PLOTINUS did not even discuss the already known fact that the visual angle enclosing an object becomes smaller with increasing distance from the object.

In summary: PLOTINUS added nothing constructive to the science of vision, since he failed to apply systematically the concepts of anatomy and optics, nor did he ever try to support his logical analysis by experiment and observation. In fact, PLOTINUS neglected the rich sources of observational material available in the optical treatises of Galen and other writers of antiquity. He failed to present the problems with the clarity which distinguished Galen's treatises from most other ancient books on optics. PLOTINUS' method of dealing with the problems of visual perception represented a noticeable decline of the empirical and experimental approach to medical science, whereas Galen had always tried to perfect his ideas by observation and experiment [295].

291 SIEGEL, *The paradoxes of Zeno* (1959).
292 PLOTINUS, *Enneades*, II, 8, 1 and 2.
293 PLOTINUS, *Enneades*, II, 8, 1.
294 PLOTINUS, *Enneades*, II, 8, 2.
295 Somewhat later another treatise on optical perception was written by DAMIANUS who probably lived during the 4th century A.D. (SARTON, Introduction, vol. 1, p. 354). Its title is *Heliodorou Larissaiou kephalaia ton optikon*; it was edited as: *Damianos, Schrift über Optik*, by R. SCHOENE, Berlin, 1897. DAMIANUS repeated mainly geometrical ideas of visual perception without referring to Galen, but mentioned PLATO, PTOLEMY and HERO. He stated that the light which originated in the pupil is similar to sunlight; that it splits up into separate lightrays on its way to the object; that it forms a rectangular discontinuous cone; that we see mainly by the moving central rays and estimate size by the visual angle. Color is added during reflection from the surface of the object. Physiological discussions, as those of Galen, are missing.

CONCLUSION: RESOLUTION OF THE LOGICAL IMPASSE

For a long time Galen's twofold approach, the geometric and the pneumatic analysis of visual perception, played a predominant role, although most later scientists and philosophers rarely referred to him. It appears remarkable that they frequently searched for a compromise between his two views in order to overcome the contradiction already discussed in the preceding analysis of Galen's doctrine of vision. Since the study of the optical research during the post-galenic period lies beyond the purpose of this book, only few references will be given to point out that the problem and the answers remained almost unchanged for nearly 1200 years.

LINDBERG[296] explained in a recent paper that ALHAZEN (965–1039) did not interpret the Epicurean emission from the object to the observing eye as a atomic 'image' or 'skin' as modern historians suggested, but that ALHAZEN spoke rather of a transfer of 'powers' and 'qualitative changes'. This idea was explained before (p. 22) as Galen's own opinion. Another scientist of the 9th and 10th century A.D., AVICEBRON, spoke likewise of the Epicurean emission as 'of powers and rays flowing forth ...' Furthermore ROGER BACON (1214–1294) supported this view when he wrote that 'this power is called likeness, image or species and is designated by many other names ... It acts on sense, intellect and on all the matter'. BACON even stated that, although 'species is not a body, ... form can not be separated from matter ... Rather it produces a likeness to itself in the air ... by drawing forth out ... the potentiality of the matter of air'.

Even GROSSETESTE (1175–1253) still combined the pneumatic with the optical concepts of Galen's visual doctrine, when he wrote:

> 'The visible species [issuing from the eye] is a substance, shining and radiating like the sun, the radiation of which, when joined with the radiation of the exterior shining body, entirely completes vision.'

In his conclusion LINDBERG pointed out that the medieval concept of the Epicurean species or image was not a corpuscular concept but

296 LINDBERG (1967). All quotations on this page are from LINDBERG's paper.

was derived from the idea of power. However, he did not refer to the similar statement of Galen who had stated that the Epicurean 'image' was an *alloiosis*, a change in the optical medium similar to what ARISTOTLE or the Stoics already had postulated. Galen's interpretation of the optical concept of the atomists has been analyzed in an earlier chapter of this study. This view has also evidently been accepted by some medieval scientists. It remains to be seen to which extent they combined this interpretation of the 'image' with the geometrical rules derived from the concepts of perspective and light rays.

Although KEPLER [297] established that light rays projected the image on the retina, he retained the traditional opinion about the further transmission of an orderly picture through the optic nerve to the brain, since he still believed in Galen's pneumatic type of nerve conduction.

The pneumatic concept of neural transmission ultimately became replaced by the modern theory of nerve conduction, whereas the geometrical doctrine of vision advanced through further anatomical discoveries. During the last century the optic nerve fibers could be followed from the retinal cells to the occipital area of the brain, where the sensory cortical cells were found to be arranged in such a manner that they preserved the spatial relation of the retinal cells. By this mechanism the 'image' on the retina is projected without distortion to the cells of the optical area of the brain. (We will not discuss here that due to the crossing of half of each optic nerve at the chiasma, the 'image' is projected to the brain in such a manner that only the left half of each retina is represented on the left, but the right half on the right occipital area of the brain.)

In recent years electron-microscopic studies of the ultra-structures of the eye eliminated the basic contradiction between the analysis of vision by light rays and the doctrine of nerve conduction. It has now been finally established that the light rays arrive at countless points of microscopical extension, i.e. at particles in the rods and cones of the retina, from where the stimuli travel along the innumerable microscopical fibers of the optic nerve to other similar sub-cellular units in the cerebral optical cortex. These biological elements, although of measurable dimension, approximate the galenic concept of points in

297 KEPLER discovered the exact point-to-point projection of the image on the retina, whereas PLATTER (1583), spoke only of the retina as sensitive visual receptor. For details of the historical development, see CROMBIE (1967).

the eye and of lines along which the optical impression was supposed to travel through the optic nerve.

It has furthermore been established that a single light ray stimulates, by the impact of one single light-quantum, a sensory subunit in the light-receptive cells of the eye [298]. Thus, a correlation between the purely physical event of light transmission and the physiological doctrine of stimulation of retinal cells and nerve conduction has been established. Anatomy also has explained how the 'image' is being preserved in its original arrangement.

Since micro-analysis of the receptive parts of the retina has established that the sensory points of the eye are responding to single light rays and that the nerve fibers approximate the lines of rays which Galen postulated between eye and brain, a satisfactory approximation between the anatomical and geometrical aspects of vision has been found, with the result that we can relate optical conduction to physiological processes without contradiction. Thus, modern research was ultimately able to eliminate the traditional and almost insuperable contradiction between the geometrical and pneumatic aspects of vision which Galen already tried to overcome.

Even if the analysis would proceed beyond the molecular structure, the transfer of the biological event to the state of psychological awareness will never be understood, regardless whether the lens of the eye, according to ARISTOTLE, or the brain, as Galen pointed out, is the principal sensory organ. Galen's statement that the cerebral pneuma represented the 'instrument of the soul' applies equally to the physicochemical forces of the cerebral structures. Galen had defined with great clarity the conceptual limits of physiological research of sense perception.

298 HUBBARD and KROPF (1967).

II. STRUCTURE AND FUNCTION OF THE AUDITORY ORGAN

A. GALEN'S DESCRIPTION OF THE INNER EAR (Figure 9)

It appears likely that Galen studied the anatomy of the ear of the ox or other large animals but never dissected the human ear. However, we know today that the sensory parts of the inner ear appear to be quite similar in ox and man. In most animals, the eardrum covers the cavity of the middle ear and conducts the acoustic vibrations through the small bones, which were still unknown to Galen, to the inner ear deep in the petrous bone. We know further that auditory perception takes place in the cochlea *(helix)* of the inner ear. The fibers of the acoustic nerves enter the petrous bone from above to be distributed throughout the membrane of the cochlea, the true acoustic end-organ. Close to it the vestibular apparatus (labyrinth) serves only as the organ of equilibrium. Both labyrinth and cochlea are filled with a clear fluid. They become visible only after the petrous bone has been cut accurately and carefully across the area of these structures.

Galen wrote that he laid open the delicate channels of the inner ear. If Galen used monkeys for this purpose, as some authors think, he must have employed magnifying lenses. But he stated that he was able to observe in the ox many structures too small to be seen in the human body. It has not yet been proved whether the ancients were familiar with the technique of preparing even primitive lenses, although evidence exists of the occasional use of such tools in engraving. There is some likelihood that curved semiprecious stones, found in a natural state, served for enlargement. But Galen never spoke of their use.

Galen investigated the anatomy of the inner ear less thoroughly than that of the eye, since he failed to consider the ear drum as responsible for perception. He attributed this function exclusively to the parts situated deep in the petrous bone. ARISTOTLE had never given a specific name to the eardrum, but he knew it, and described its great vulnerability. He even mentioned that the eardrum bursts when a diver reaches deep water, and that sponges attached to the outside of the ear could prevent the rupture of the drum under the increased water pressure. In this context, ARISTOTLE simply spoke of the 'ear' *(ota)*[1]. Likewise, Galen referred only briefly to the 'cover' *(skepasma)* of the external ear canal but did not employ any specific anatomical term for the ear drum.

Furthermore, Galen did not believe that this covering membrane *(skepasma)* could protect the inner ear. He wrote that if it would be strong enough to hold the air back, it would interfere with hearing. Without any further thought about the possible function of the ear-drum, Galen explained, on the basis of purely teleological speculation, that the best protection of the acoustic nerve against injury was its position deep in the solid petrous bone. Galen wrote that, for this purpose, the 'ear canal' narrowed gradually from its external opening to the spirally shaped organ of the inner ear (*helix*, spiral). This arrangement seemed to him 'created' not only for reducing the impact of air vibrations on the deeply imbedded acoustic nerve but also for protecting the ear from accidentally entering foreign bodies. Likewise, cold air would be prevented from reaching these inner recesses, since otherwise it could easily damage the sensory nerve or the adjacent part of the brain[2].

Galen also failed to describe the anatomical and functional features of the cavity and the small bones (ossicles) of the middle ear, since

1 ARISTOTLE, *Problemata* XXXII; 1, 2, 11. The importance of this statement does not change if one considers the *Problemata* as the work of ARISTOTLE's successor.
2 DAREMBERG, vol. 1, p. 546; KUEHN, vol. 3, p. 643ff.; Galen, *De usu partium*, book 8, chap. 6.

Figure 9. Structures of the human ear[1].

This drawing represents a cross-section of the human ear. Galen knew the external ear canal, the drum and the helix of the inner ear which is located in the petrous bone. However, he failed to describe the cavity of the middle ear with its small bones, which conduct the sound waves from the drum to the fluid-filled *helix*, the receptive organ of the inner ear. He also did not recognize the importance of the vestibular apparatus of the inner ear for the maintenance of equilibrium. But he described the course of the facial nerve through the petrous bone around the inner ear.
Galen thought that the sound waves of the air were transmitted by the air directly from the external ear canal to the *helix* of the inner ear in which the acoustic nerve terminates. He regarded the eardrum only as a membrane protecting the deeper structures.

1 This drawing is a reproduction of figure 1 of MAX BROEDEL's *Three unpublished drawings of the anatomy of the human ear* (Saunders, Philadelphia 1946) with the permission of the publishing house.

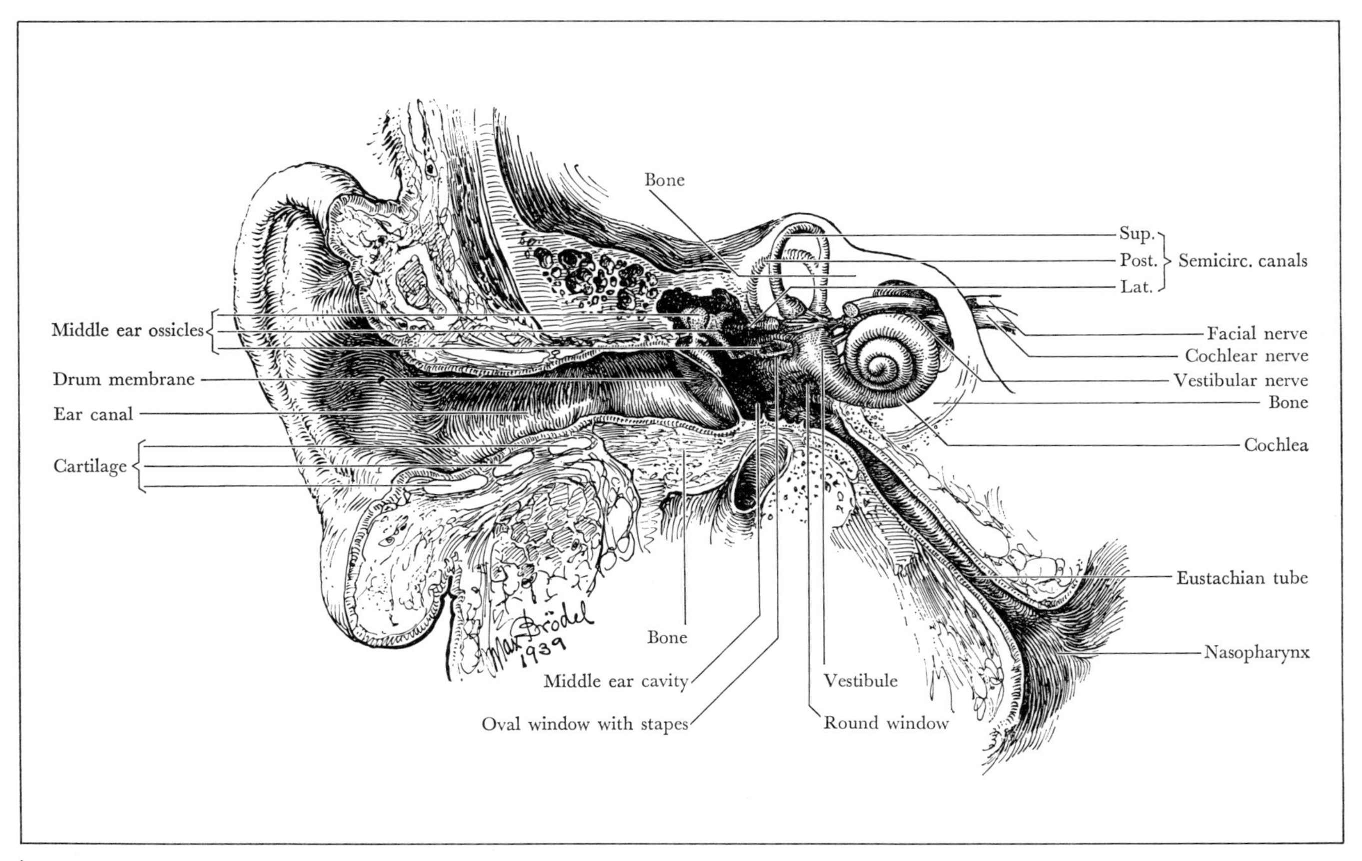
Sup.
Post.
Lat.
Semicirc. canals
Facial nerve
Cochlear nerve
Vestibular nerve
Bone
Cochlea
Eustachian tube
Nasopharynx
Bone
Vestibule
Round window
Bone
Middle ear cavity
Oval window with stapes
Middle ear ossicles
Drum membrane
Ear canal
Cartilage

he outlined only the structures of the external ear canal and inner ear. He wrote:

> 'Nature has placed a kind of spiral-shaped labyrinth through a slanting perforation [of the external ear-canal] in the dense and hard [petrous] bone.' [2]

Galen was convinced that in the narrow ear canal the soundwaves (see p. 132) gradually lose their intensity until they come in contact with the terminal fibers of the acoustic nerve. He correctly observed that this nerve spreads out in the helix of the ear like the optic nerve in the retina (p. 56).

It has often been questioned whether Galen actually described the inner ear and it has been even denied that he called the inner ear 'labyrinth'. WERNER even wrote that Galen called the external ear-canal 'labyrinth'. The present study of the Greek text revealed, however, that Galen's terminology was not ambiguous. First of all, he stated that the outer ear-canal is not as tortuous as the cochlea but only slightly curved, often even straight. He also called the ear lobe *konchion, (conchula)* but not labyrinth. The Latin term *concha* indicated a mussel with a bivalvular shell *(konchion)* and *conchula* is its diminutive form. Mussels are flat and almost shaped as the outer ear. Secondly, several passages in his treatises proved that Galen did actually demonstrate the delicate structures of the inner ear in the petrous bone. These he called *helix (cochlea)*. The spiral cavity of the acoustic end-organ still bears this name which admirably describes its shape: it has a comparatively wide entrance but narrows to the end point like the shell of certain snails. Galen stated that he studied the structures of the ear by chipping away gradually the hard petrous bone in order to demonstrate the acoustic organ. He was also able to separate the auditory structures from the tortuous canal through which the facial nerve passes toward the base of the skull. He wrote:

> 'If one cuts off slowly the whole bone and frees the nerve, then the coils [*helikes*] at its end can be demonstrated, and the [facial] nerve which penetrates near the ear to the outside.' [3]

2 KUEHN, vol. 8, p. 844.

3 Galen repeatedly pointed out that the facial nerve passes along a narrow winding canal (canalis Falloppii of modern terminology) which surrounds partly the

In this passage, DAREMBERG translated *helix* erroneously as 'detour'. Thus he failed to realize that Galen indeed discovered the internal acoustic organ.

The meaning of the term 'labyrinth' in Galen's writings has now to be defined. We call the three small vestibular canals of the organ of equilibrium in the petrous bone by the name 'labyrinth'. But Galen apparently did not consider a separate function of the vestibular canals, nor did he visualize these as separate structures. He simply indicated by the name *labyrinthos* the entire assembly of minute cavities in the petrous bone as far as he was able to demonstrate without the aid of the sophisticated methods of later periods. Galen used the term *labyrinthos* likewise to describe the vascular coils of the testicle or the rete mirabilis, even the small crisscrossing paths of anthills were called *labyrinth*[4].

Galen described that the acoustic nerve terminated in the *helix* of the inner ear in a manner comparable to the fanning out of the optic nerve in the retina:

> 'For the same reason as in the eye the optic nerve spreads into the lens, the [acoustic] nerve spreads at the inner end of the ear-canal, where its fibers flatten out to attach themselves [to the helix]. Past this canal, all parts [of the acoustic nerve] spread over the spiral convolutions of the helix in the same manner as [the optic nerve spreads through the retinal fibers into] the lens of the eye.'[5]

As mentioned before, Galen obviously overlooked the cavity and the ossicles of the middle ear, since he wrote that the external ear-canal comes to an end at the sensory structures of the [inner] ear in the petrous bone (fig. 9).

He was further convinced that the inner ear served only as an acoustic organ, since he did not associate the maintenance of equilibrium with the function of these osseous canals.

---

acoustic organ in the petrous bone. Galen described further the facial peri-orbital muscles derived from the 5th and 7th nerves (modern numeration). Since these structures are not related to hearing, further details will be omitted. Galen, *De usu partium*, lib. 9, chap. 10; KUEHN, vol. 3, p. 724; DAREMBERG, vol. 1, p. 589.

4 LIDDELL-SCOTT, Greek-English Dictionary (1958).

5 KUEHN, vol. 7, p. 103.

B. GALEN'S DOCTRINE OF SOUND AND SOUND PERCEPTION

Galen discussed two possibilities of how the sensory structures of the inner ear could be stimulated by the incoming sound. When formulating his doctrine of transmission of a visual impression to the optic nerve Galen had decided in favor of the transfer of the optical image by changes passing through a pneumatic medium in space, but refuted the concept of a material transfer of the image as impossible [6]. For the doctrine of hearing, the same alternative arose whether we are dealing with transmission of the acoustic stimulus through stationary air (by propagation of sound waves) or with a flow of air.

As in all the other fields, Galen's ideas were deeply rooted in traditional concepts. Before we analyze his views, we have to discuss whether his predecessors were familiar with the concept of propagation of sound waves.

Long before Galen, the ancient philosophers had debated whether sound was propagated through space by vibration of the air. ARISTOTLE compared the advance of sound through air to the propagation of a visual impression through the 'transparent' medium. He stated that air does not flow from the source of sound to the ear but that a change in the structure of the air, characteristic of each sound, moves rapidly toward the auditory organ. ARISTOTLE wrote further that the ear contained 'air' *(pneuma)* but failed to clarify whether this was outside air or a pneuma generated in the body itself:

> 'The medium of sound is air.' [7]
> 'The air in the ear always moves according to a motion of its own.' [8]
> 'The so-called empty space *(kenon)* [of the inner parts of the ear] is full of air *(aer)*.' [9]

But ARISTOTLE did not consider a vacuum in our modern sense when he wrote that the inner ear is 'empty':

6 See chapter on vision, p. 49ff.
7 ARISTOTLE, *De anima*, 419 a 34.
8 ARISTOTLE, *On the soul*, 420 a 17.
9 ARISTOTLE, *On the soul*, 419 b 34; BEARE, p. 114 (1906).

'Air is commonly thought to be empty [space].'
'Kenon einai dokei ho aer'.[10]

The Greek word *kenon*, empty, has often been erroneously translated as vacuum, a term which evidently gives a distorted view of ARISTOTLE's doctrine. Like the ancients, ARISTOTLE used the term 'empty' without thinking of a true vacuum[10].

Like ARISTOTLE, Galen did not consider the inner ear as a vacuum but he declared that it is filled with air. Galen denied that a flow of air could penetrate the gradually narrowing channel of the petrous bone toward the sensory organ of hearing. Therefore, he agreed with ARISTOTLE that sound was propagated only by the advance of some subtle change in the air, but not by a current of air. This description obviously implied an undulatory movement of the air. ARISTOTLE had already described this wave motion of the air but without using the term 'wave':

> 'In order to survive an animal should not only have perception by immediate contact but also from afar . . . through a sensory medium which is affected by the object, but which in turn affects the animal. For exactly as that [event] which has produced a motion on one spot by inducing changes, thus this impulse *(to osan)* elicits another impulse and, therefore, a motion will take place through a medium: that which moved first impels without itself being impelled . . . There are different media, as it seems. But the effect of alteration *(alloiosis)* [of the medium] is that an object can produce a change while remaining on the same spot.'[11]

10 ARISTOTLE, *On the soul*, 419 b 33; also *Parts of animals*, 656 b 17.—ARISTOTLE believed that the ear is connected with the brain through a channel *(poros)* filled with air. His argument was based, as CLARKE explained, on the observation in some animals of a large endolymphatic sac leading from the inner ear to the posterior part of the brain. Furthermore, he believed that in the turtle the brain appeared to be smaller than the cavity of the skull, since on dissection the occiput was partly empty. ARISTOTLE, therefore, seemed to think that the outside air was connected with the air in the skull behind the brain (ARISTOTLE, *Parts of animals*, II, 10 (Loeb ed., p. 177); CLARKE, J. Hist. Med. allied Sci. (1963), expressed astonishment at this statement, since ARISTOTLE located conscious sense perception in the heart to which the acoustic stimulus was supposedly conducted through the blood stream.—Galen often used the word *pneuma* as synonymous with the air we inhale. When a specific pneuma was considered he usually added the words *zotikon* or *psychikon*.

11 ARISTOTLE, *On the soul*, 434 b 26 – 435 a 4; BEARE translated the text of ARISTOTLE: 'Sound alters the air', but one should preferably translate the Greek term

Shortly after ARISTOTLE but still long before Galen, ZENO, the founder of the Stoic school of philosophy (3rd century B.C.) had expressed an even more definite opinion on wave-motion:

> 'We hear when the air between the sonant body and the organ of hearing suffers a concussion, a vibration, which spreads spherically and then forms waves and strikes upon the ears, just as water in a reservoir forms circles when a stone is thrown into it.' [12]

ZENO indeed employed here the word *kyma*, wave.

In his own studies, Galen did not simply follow ARISTOTLE's concept, but he discussed the two possible modes of motion of air: sound could be perceived either when an advancing column of air reached the ear, or by the impact of air-waves on the acoustic end-organ. Only the second idea seemed to correspond to ARISTOTLE's concept of sound or light passing through a stationary medium. Galen wrote:

> 'In regard to hearing, an outgrowth [the acoustic nerve] of the brain has to descend in order to receive a stimulus arriving from the outside. When this is a tone or a noise, the air has either to be stricken *(aer peplegmenos)* [producing a flow of air] or a stroke

---

'*he phone aer tis eschatismenos*' as: 'Sound is air which has taken up a specific shape'. In modern terms this would indicate that sound waves have a particular length according to the pitch of the tone. (BEARE, p. 116, note 1, referring to ARISTOTLE, *Problemata*, XI, 904 b 27). (My own translation.)

12 DIOGENES LAERTIUS, VII, No. 158.—EPICURUS, a philosopher almost contemporary with ARISTOTLE, explained the propagation of sound as a flow of air, since this seemed to derive from the atomic doctrine. He, therefore, postulated that sound traveled as a stream (*rheuma*, from *rheo*, flow) of air particles. However, he tried to visualize how 'air itself' was molded by the voice. He thought that a 'certain interconnection of the particles of the air' was preserved. As in the doctrine of vision, a pattern had to be maintained by the atoms which ordinarily moved at random. This additional postulate was, to a certain degree, alien to the atomistic doctrine. Furthermore, EPICURUS spoke of a definite connection *(sympatheia)* of the part when he wrote:

> 'Without the transfer of such a *sympathy*, the auditory sense perception could not take place.'

The term *sympathy* indicated the response to the pattern which was maintained during the transmission of the stimulus (DIOGENES LAERTIUS, X, 52–53). Thus, as in the doctrine of vision (p. 17ff.), the atomistic and Aristotelian ideas were not as completely antagonistic as mostly assumed.

(plexis) has to become a condition of the air *(plexis this hyparchousa aeros)* [i.e. the air becomes a stationary medium of waves], unless both are the same. The motion of this impact *(plege)* should proceed like a wave *(kyma)* upwards to the brain.'[13]

Galen did not mention whether he undertook experiments to clarify this issue. But it is likely that the concept of sound-waves had already become the accepted doctrine of the propagation of acoustic impressions. Most of the relevant treatises of the Hellenistic period have been lost. However, the later literature does not seem to be much different from the earlier discussions. Thus, we read in a treatise of PHILOPONOS of the 6th century A.D.:

'If we pass a wet finger around the rim of a glass filled with water, a sound is created by the air squeezed out by the finger. This air is ejected into the cavity of the cup producing the sound by striking against the walls . . . If one fills a cup with water, we can see how ripples are produced in the water when the finger moves around the rim. Obviously, the air ejected by the pressure of the finger creates the motion of the water.'[14]

BOETHIUS, a Roman statesman and author of the 5th century A.D., stated in a similar manner:

'In the case of sound, something of the same sort takes place as when a stone is thrown out and falls into a pool or other calm water. The stone first produces a wave with a very small circumference; then it causes the waves to spread out in ever wider circles until the motion, growing weaker as the waves spread out, finally ceases.'[15]

Thus, the concept of propagation of sound by waves must have been quite familiar to the scientists of Galen's time, regardless whether the medium was air or water. Evidently, Galen had failed to recognize that the delicate canals of the inner ear were filled with a clear watery fluid (called today endolymph). This mistake confirmed him further

13 KUEHN, vol. 3, p. 644ff.
14 SAMBURSKI, p. 100 (1962).
15 COHEN and DRABKIN, p. 293.

in the concept of *pneuma* as the basis of sound perception. Galen, however, did not commit the error of the philosophers to speak of a preexisting, 'innate' or 'connate' pneuma *(emphyton pneuma)* as recipient of sound in the inner ear, but he considered the air *(pneuma)* in the sensory part of the ear as identical with the outside air[16].

Although Galen presented a reasonable physical explanation for the transfer of sound to the acoustic nerve, he had failed to answer the question of how the vibration of air was transferred to the brain. It seemed as if the problem could be explained by postulating that the sound waves caused a corresponding stimulus to the 'air' present in the sensory nerve. However, Galen did not state that the acoustic nerve contained air in the physical sense, when he stipulated that all nerves were activated by the cerebral pneuma (p. 73, referring to *dynamis*, power).

Galen remained ambiguous about the nature of this *cerebral pneuma*, speaking of its gas-like nature, to use a modern expression, but at the same time considering it as imponderable[16]. It remained, therefore, questionable how the acoustic vibrations could reach the sensory area of the cerebral ventricles which were supposedly filled with the cerebral pneuma.

When Galen did not see a clear answer he often lost himself in teleological speculations which, as in this instance, were hardly worth repeating. But the oversight of the ossicles in the middle ear and the pneumatic doctrine of nerve conduction were the two principal stumbling blocks to further progress of Galen's doctrine of acoustic perception.

Again and again Galen tried to convince his contemporaries that the brain was the seat of perception and thought. It was difficult to convince them of the errors of traditional ideas. As previously mentioned, PLATO and ARISTOTLE projected the conscious seat of sensation into the liver or heart. According to their doctrine, the perceived sound was transferred, in an unexplained manner, by the pneuma and the blood to these organs (see also footnote 10). Galen, however, clearly defined conscious perception as an activity of the brain. The propagation of the acoustic stimulus through the acoustic nerve into the cerebral ventricles corresponded therefore to Galen's general pattern of perception.

16 The problem of pneuma has been discussed in detail in SIEGEL, p. 414 (1968), where extensive references are cited. ARISTOTLE thought that air or *pneuma* could be present in the ear before birth, like the pneuma in the nervous system. ARISTOTLE, *De generatione animalium*, II, 6: 744 a 3; see also p. 65.

C. HUMORS AND DISEASES OF THE EAR

We know today that the so-called Eustachian tube leads from the middle ear to the pharynx. Although it has chiefly the function of maintaining normal air pressure in the middle ear, it also might serve as outflow-tract for secretions. ARISTOTLE, who already had recognized the existence of this tube, did not realize that it leads into the middle ear. He attributed to it only the function of carrying superfluous matter from the inner ear to the oral cavity. He wrote that there was no passage from the *stromboi* (spiral-shell, i.e., the *helix* of the inner ear; see p. 129) to the brain, but that he had found an outlet leading cerebral waste to the roof of the mouth[17].

Galen failed to mention this tube when he discussed that the brain discharged superfluous matter through nose and palate, since he mostly spoke of seepage passing from both the infundibulum and the pituitary gland toward the nasal and oral cavities (p. 147). But he considered serous or purulent drainage from the brain via the external auditory canal as feasible, although he must have assumed that it would have to pass through the narrow channels of the inner ear. Likewise, drugs applied to the ear were thought to penetrate deeply via the drum through the inner ear into the petrous bone[18].

Galen stated that acoustic perception can be damaged at three anatomical locations: in the area of the brain where the auditory nerves originated, in the acoustic nerve, and finally, in the ear itself[19]. Although he did not support this statement by clinical description of pertinent cases, Galen explained the often fatal outcome of acute earache as a penetration of 'humors' into the brain. We know today that these cases were most likely caused by acute infections of the middle ear, when accumulated pus was able to penetrate through the bone into meninges[20]. Ear-wax was understood as a harmless secretion of the brain[21].

Galen classified the diseases of the ear according to the various humoral disturbances which cannot be discussed here, since interest-

17 ARISTOTLE, *Hist. anim.*, 492 a 20.
18 KUEHN, vol. 10, p. 455.
19 KUEHN, vol. 7, p. 102.
20 KUEHN, vol. 18 b, p. 261, 262.
21 KUEHN, vol. 17 b, p. 240. For a detailed analysis of Galen's description of diseases of the ear, see POLITZER.

ing clinical material became unintelligible by his rather unattractive and difficult terminology. Only one syndrome should be discussed since Galen attributed it to a disturbance of humors or pneuma in the ear. Today we know, however, that it is mostly caused by an affection of the vestibular nerve or its end-organ in the petrous bone.

D. DESCRIPTION OF DIZZINESS (MENIÈRE'S DISEASE)

The following text is a translation of a passage from Galen's treatise *On the diseased organs* which presented the syndrome nowadays known as MENIÈRE's disease. It should be mentioned in advance that the Greek word *skotoma* could mean both dizziness and darkness (*skotos*, dark). Galen considered both fainting and blurring of normal vision as an important manifestation of a humoral disturbance. He wrote:

> 'All these affections start obviously in the head and especially the affection which is called *skotoma* (vertigo), the name of which indicates its nature. People who are subject to this ailment are affected by *skotoma* of their vision on account of the smallest causes, so that they often fall, especially when they turn around. Then, what happens to other people only after having turned around a great many times, that will overcome these people after one single turn. They can even be affected by vertigo, when they see another person or a wheel turning or anything else which whirls, even when they see the whirling motion in the river. These people are still more liable to such an attack when they have been exposed to the sun or when their head had been overheated for any other reason ... There is agreement upon the fact that such frequent turning movements provoke an unequal, tumultuous and disorderly flow of humors and pneuma. Therefore, it is only natural that people subject to skotoma are on guard against any motion of this kind.
>
> It has been proved that relief is obtained by cutting the artery. One has to incise deeply and piece by piece the arteries situated behind the ear, to such an extent that a deep scar is created between the two separated sections. But it is also sure that not all cases can be cured by this procedure, because there still are other arteries of more considerable size than the latter which rise from

the base of the skull to the brain or from the retiform plexus *(rete mirabilis)*. It is quite plausible that these arteries can cause the same syndrome, when a vaporous and warm pneuma, rising through these arteries, fills the brain. It is also possible that in the brain itself a dyscrasia is produced, when a similar pneuma is generated ... This can result in an obvious black-out of the sensory perception. This can be both a primary disease of the head or, on occasion a sympathetic disease arising from an affection of the cavity of the stomach.

ARCHIGENES described likewise these facts in his first book *The pathognomonic signs of chronic diseases*, when he spoke of a spell of vertigo *(skotoma)* in the following terms: "This affection has two causes, either in the head or in the hypochondria." Then, he attempted to distinguish the two kinds by saying that vertigo represented a primary affection of the head preceded by ringing of the ears, pain and heaviness in the head, or a disturbance of the sense of smell and damage of the sensory parts originating there ... He further stated that, when vertigo originates in the cavity of the stomach, it is preceeded by pain in the cardia *(kardiogmos)* and nausea. As I myself have stated previously more than once, we have to realize that, even if the head suffers by sympathetic affection related to another organ, it is still the head to which we have to attribute the symptoms as they appear.' [22]

This description is typical of what we now call MENIÈRE's disease which is the result of an affection of the inner ear, especially of the vestibular branch of the 8th nerve (modern term) or of the organ of equilibrium, the vestibular canals (modern term). Although Galen did not know the difference between the vestibular and the acoustic parts of the fifth nerve (his numeration), his clinical description of the syndrome was adequate. Galen unknowingly anticipated a vascular interpretation of this syndrome i.e. a disturbance of the blood flow through the arteries of the ear, since he recommended cutting the arteries supplying this area in the endeavor to divert abnormal humors. It would, however, be wrong to say that Galen recognized the circulatory cause of this disease, although clinical intuition led him to correct localization of this syndrome.

22 DAREMBERG, vol. 2, pp. 574–576; Galen, *De locis affertis*, book 3, chap. 12; KUEHN, vol. 8, pp. 201–204. Also, discussion on sympathy, SIEGEL, pp. 360–382 (1968). SKOTOMA reminds of the expression 'black-out'.

III. STRUCTURE AND FUNCTION OF THE OLFACTORY ORGAN

A. ANATOMY OF THE PERIPHERAL AND CENTRAL ORGANS OF SMELL (Figure 10, 11)

We encounter two difficulties in understanding Galen's doctrine of olfactory perception: firstly, his description of the organ of smell was based only on dissection of animals; secondly, he derived his doctrine of smell from the pneumatic concept of nervous activity.

Galen's detailed description of the anatomy of the external structures of the nose[1] can be omitted as unimportant for his doctrine of sense perception. Whereas modern anatomists count the olfactory nerve as the first of the twelve cranial nerves, we shall see that Galen was indeed correct when he considered the olfactory structures not as true cranial nerves but as part of the brain itself. Consisting of the olfactory bulb and trunk this organ seemed to have a double duty: perception

1 Galen, *De usu partium*, book 9, chap. 17; DAREMBERG, vol. 1, p. 695; KUEHN, vol. 3, p. 918.

Figure 10. Schematic view of the human olfactory apparatus (lateral view).

Both the olfactory tract and bulb are situated above the dura mater, below the frontal lobe of the brain. From the olfactory bulb numerous sensory fibers penetrate first the dura mater, then the lamina cribrosa, the sieve-like membrane of the ethmoidal bone between the cavity of the skull and the nasal cavity. The sensory olfactory fibers terminate in the upper (shaded) area of the nasal cavity. Galen failed to observe these fibers. He described, however, in domestic animals a cavity in the olfactory bulb which communicates through a slender canal in the olfactory tract with the cerebral ventricles, the assumed seat of cerebral pneuma (spiritus animalis).The cavity of the bulb and the canal in the tract are not indicated in this drawing.
Galen thought that odoriferous substances travel with inhaled air from the nasal cavity into the olfactory bulb whereas mucus or purulent discharges take this course in the reverse direction from the bulb to the nasal cavity. Thus the olfactory bulb was thought to be both a sensory and an excretory organ.

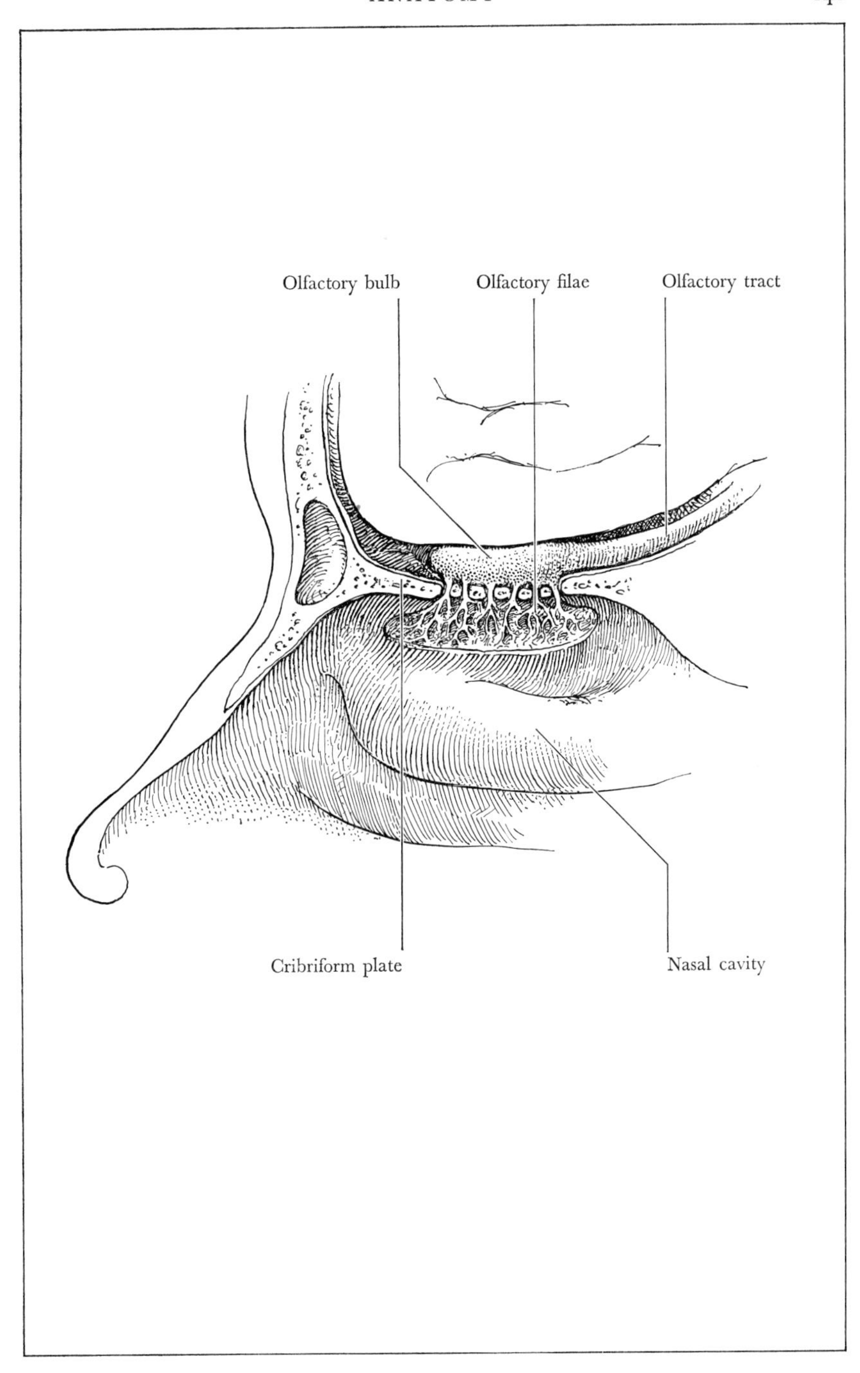
Olfactory bulb
Olfactory filae
Olfactory tract
Cribriform plate
Nasal cavity

and awareness of odors, and excretion of metabolic residues from the brain and its cavities [2].

We know today that only the uppermost part of the nasal mucosa, close to the base of the skull, contains cells sensitive to odors. They send the stimuli through the fila olfactoria to the olfactory bulb. Galen, however, did not consider any part of the nasal cavity as sensitive to odor, since he regarded the nasal channels and the pores in their roof only as passages leading to a sense organ at a higher level. The reasons for Galen's error were based on misinterpretation of anatomical findings and on concepts derived from the pneumatic doctrine of nerve conduction and brain action.

Galen's idea was that the odors travel as very fine particles [3] from the nasal cavity through openings in the lamina cribrosa of the ethmoid and the adjacent 'pores' of the nasal and meningeal membranes into the olfactory area of the brain (bulbus olfactorius).

Galen thought that he could demonstrate on animals which just had died that the nasal mucosa was pierced by numerous perforations which were situated opposite to the pores of the lamina cribrosa. These openings could only be seen after stretching the detached nasal membrane or by pouring hot water over it. In extreme cold or a long time after death these fine apertures, hidden in the deep folds of the mucous membrane, seemed to become invisible by contraction [4].

Galen correctly described that the nasal cavity is separated from the cavity of the skull by the horizontal extension of the ethmoid bone which bears the name *lamina cribrosa*, the sieve-like plate (*ethmos*, strainer, in Latin, *cribrum*). We know that numerous small openings in this thin plate permit the sensory fibers of the olfactory organ to enter the upper

2 A diagram of these structures is presented in figures 4, 10 and 11 of this treatise and in SIEGEL, fig. 7, p. 119 (1968).

3 KUEHN, vol. 2, p. 862; *leptomeres*, composed of small particles.

4 DAREMBERG, vol. 1, p. 548; Galen, *De usu partium*, book 8, chap. 6; KUEHN, vol. 3, p. 648.

Figure 11. Olfactory system of the horse (lateral view, schematic drawing).

The olfactory tract connects the large olfactory bulb to the anterior part of the brain. The olfactory bulb has a narrow ventricle which communicates through a slender canal of its tract with the cerebral ventricles. The olfactory bulb also sends nerve fibers to the nasal cavity which are not shown in this drawing but in Fig. 10. They were unknown to Galen. The cavities in bulb and tract are not shown in this drawing.

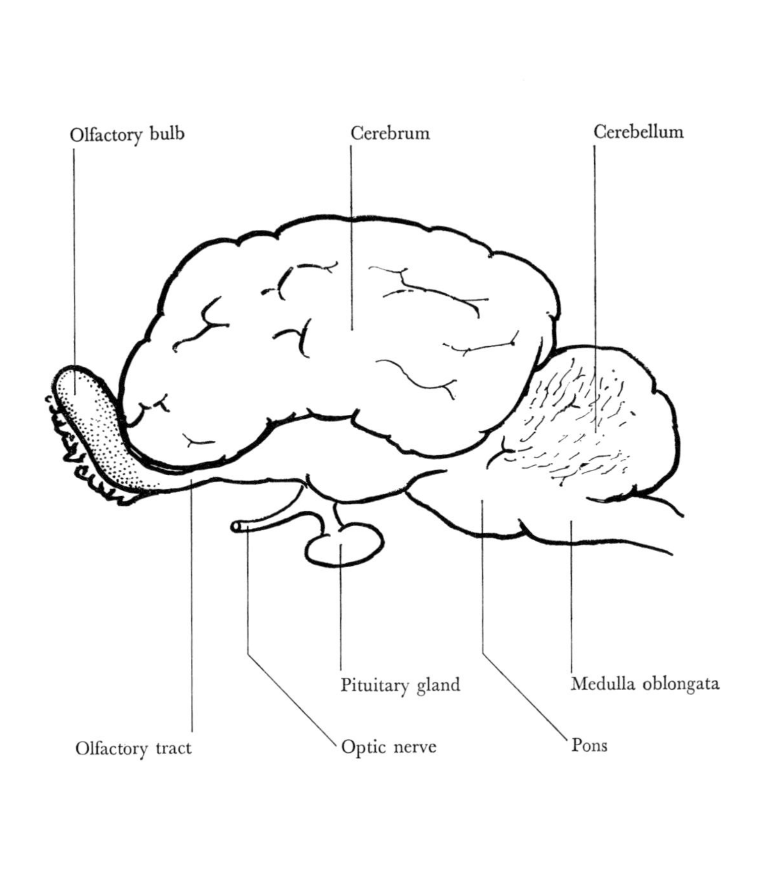
Olfactory bulb
Cerebrum
Cerebellum
Pituitary gland
Medulla oblongata
Olfactory tract
Optic nerve
Pons

area of the nasal cavity (Fig. 10). But Galen, failing to detect these delicate nerve fibers connecting the olfactory bulb with the nasal mucosa *(filae olfactoriae)*, did not believe in a complete separation of the two cavities.

Galen recommended the exchange of the term sieve-like bone *(ethmoid)* for the more descriptive expression *spongoid* which HIPPOCRATES had already proposed because of the greater thickness of the part of the ethmoid bone nearer the pituitary gland and its irregular structural pattern. Conduits seemed to lead in curved lines through the ethmoid bone from the nose anteriorly to the olfactory bulb, posteriorly toward the pituitary and infundibulum as drainage for metabolic residue of the brain (see p. 150). They appeared comparable to the channels of a sponge, enhancing the discharge of waste products while odors ascend. However, the term *ethmoid* is still accepted by modern anatomists.

Galen observed further the dura mater, lying above the ethmoid bone and separating it from the olfactory organ of the brain. As known to Galen already, the dura mater envelopes the entire brain and spinal cord. When Galen stretched the meningeal membrane after removal from the skull he could see, against a strong light, numerous small openings which he interpreted as continuation of the pathways of odors which had already passed through the nasal mucosa and the ethmoid bone[5]. It seemed that the pores of the dura were directly adjacent to the perforations of the *lamina cribrosa* (Fig. 10). The meningeal pores were, of course, artefacts; but Galen was unaware of his error.

Galen was further confirmed in his concept that the delicate particles of odors (see p. 142) enter directly from the nasal cavity into the olfactory bulb, when he observed that only some slender branches of the third nerve (Galen's numeration) entered the nasal cavity to terminate in the mucosal lining. (This nerve is according to modern nomenclature a part of the maxillary branch of the trigeminal nerve, the fifth of our, the third of Galen's count.) He thought that such a thin nerve could hardly qualify for the perception of odors, especially when compared to the thickness of the acoustic or optic nerve[6]. These nerve fibers also did not spread out as a terminal network[7] like the

5 DUCKWORTH, *Anatomy*, p. 5.
6 KUEHN, vol. 2, pp. 864–866.
7 Galen found that only one small branch of the trigeminal nerve supplied the nose and the upper part of the palate (DUCKWORTH, p. 194). He recognized it as part of the maxillary branch of the third nerve; Galen, *De usu partium*, book 9, chap. 8; also book 9, chap. 16; DAREMBERG, vol. 1, pp. 584, 601; KUEHN, vol. 3, pp. 712, 746 ff.

optic nerve in the retina or the auditory nerve in the *helix* (cochlea) of the inner ear. Therefore Galen came to the conclusion that the nasal branches of the maxillary nerve transmit only the sensation of touch from the interior of the nose, similar to other parts of the third nerve[8].

In conclusion, Galen did not think that there existed a peripheral end-organ for smell, as the eye for light, or the ear for sound, but that the odors were perceived directly by the olfactory brain itself. This concept was, at least, not in contradiction with his general doctrine that conscious sense perception takes place in the brain or its ventricles:

> 'The brain is the perceptive organ for the [peripheral] sense organs (*egkephalos organon . . . aithetikon aisthetikos*) and therefore sends out its perceptive power through the nerves to all parts of the organism.'[9]

Galen's artificial overstretching of the membranes and his failure to observe the delicate olfactory fibers passing through the 'sieve' of the ethmoid bone was not the only reason for assuming that the perception of smell was the function of the brain. He derived a second important reason from the study of the olfactory organ itself. These concepts were the result of animal dissection. Although Galen had made it clear that he mostly dissected animals, he has been severely criticized by those who implied that he only referred to human anatomy in his treatises on dissection.

We know today that the two principal parts which compose the olfactory organ of man, the olfactory tract and bulb, appear hardly comparable with those of domestic animals. In many animals we encounter above the lamina cribrosa of the ethmoidal bone an olfactory bulb of such considerable size that it impresses the observer as a small brain in itself (Fig. 11). The olfactory bulb is connected to the main part of the brain by a large band of nervous tissue which constitutes the olfactory tract. In some domestic animals the center of each olfactory bulb contains a cavity (olfactory ventricle) which extends as a canal through the length of the olfactory tract to the anterior cerebral ventricle of the same side (see Fig. 10, 11):

8 DUCKWORTH, *Anatomy*, p. 194; also DAREMBERG, vol. 1, p. 601; Galen, *De usu partium*, book 9, chap. 16; KUEHN, vol. 3, p. 746.
9 KUEHN, vol. 7, p. 139.

'From the brain [i.e. the anterior part of the lateral ventricles] two long horn-like processes grow out and reach to the two nasal fossae. Besides being lengthy, these two processes are hollowed out internally by an excavation which resembles that of a tubular flute [olfactory tract], and their substance is exactly like that of the brain.' [10]

In man, the olfactory bulb is only slightly bigger than a large matchhead and has no cavity nor does a hollow channel lead through the olfactory tract to the brain. Only during fetal life a rudimental, almost microscopical olfactory ventricle can be observed which obliterates before the birth of the child [11]. Galen considered the olfactory bulb as part of the brain, since it appeared as composed of distinct layers comparable to those of the brain itself.

Based on animal dissection, Galen also distinguished correctly the olfactory structures from peripheral nerves when he wrote:

'The route from each cerebral ventricle toward the nose is a long outgrowth [of the brain: the combined olfactory tract and bulb], not different from the other cavities of the brain.' [12]

We read in Galen's anatomical treatise that he supported his idea of a communication between olfactory and cerebral ventricles by pushing a probe from the lateral cerebral ventricle through the olfactory tract into the bulb:

'Betake yourself to the part where each of the two ventricles, stretching toward the front, is narrowed. Into this part insert the head-end of a thick sound. For the place itself is wide at its commencement. When you have done that, then point the sound a little upwards, cut or tear through the part stretching itself upward, and again go gradually forward until you come to the first part of the nose, where the bone lies which the anatomists name the cribriform (*cribrum*, sieve).' [13]

10 DUCKWORTH, p. 186.

11 ARIENS-KAPPERS, p. 1451.

12 Galen, *De usu partium*, book 8, chap. 6; DAREMBERG, vol. 1, p. 543; KUEHN, vol. 3, p. 640.

13 DUCKWORTH, p. 4 (partly arranged).

This procedure suggests that the described frontal openings of the olfactory canal were artefacts. Galen thought so himself:

> 'Often indeed, when I have wished to obtain a complete knowledge of the nature of this region, have I met with no slight uncertainty ... The reason for my difficulty was that it was not possible for me to ascertain by the eye [while attempting to push a probe through the cavity of the olfactory bulb and duct] whether both [olfactory] cavities come finally to a single orifice ... or whether they are closed up and blocked ... or whether fine apertures and effluents [most likely toward the lateral ventricles] are present in the [olfactory] duct ... The very nature of things makes it necessary that the [olfactory] ducts (i.e. tracts) not be closed up, since ... mucus cannot be poured without an effluent orifice of a certain diameter. Nevertheless, it is not here my purpose to derive the knowledge of the nature of things, which I wish to understand, from analogy; for this is not the aim of anatomy ... It was not possible for me to perceive with the eye how the canals leading from the brain to the nose terminate. For the matter is, as I explained, that in this region the brain is soft.'[14]

Although Galen arrived by probing at the correct conclusion that the olfactory tracts open into the ventricles, an artefact arose evidently when he searched for the distal perforations in the olfactory bulb toward the nasal area. But in spite of his doubts, Galen was quite definite about the existence of an open communication between the olfactory bulb and the cerebral ventricles when he wrote elsewhere:

> 'The olfactory bulb is a brain-structure of which the individual parts on both sides, right and left, are united to one another in one and the same manner [i.e. by the communication between the two lateral ventricles into which each olfactory tract leads].'[15]

This communication was considered as the pathway for residues from the cerebral ventricles toward the nasal cavity, leading partly

14 DUCKWORTH, *Anatomy*, p. 14; SIMON, vol. 2, p. 4.

15 DUCKWORTH, p. 5. See also Galen, *De usu partium*, book 9, chap. 1; DAREMBERG, vol. 1, p. 569 ff. See also footnote 22.

through the olfactory organ, partly through the pituitary which was supposed to drain the lateral ventricles (i.e. the third ventricles of the brain. See also p. 150).

In my own experience, it was practically impossible to dissect the ox brain a few hours after death after it had been removed from the skull by the butcher. I could, therefore, not repeat Galen's procedure. But I checked the anatomy of the olfactory structures of domestic animals in books on veterinary anatomy. Galen's outline of the olfactory organ corresponds quite well to the description in a modern text book of the olfactory anatomy of the horse[16]:

> 'The olfactory bulb is an oval enlargement which curves upward in front of the frontal pole of the hemisphere [from which it is separated]. Its convex superficial face fits into the ethmoidal fossa [of the lamina cribrosa] and receives numerous olfactory nerve-fibers (fila olfactoria) through the cribriform plate. Hence, it is very difficult to remove the bulb intact [since the fila olfactoria are torn]. It contains a considerable cavity, the ventricle of the olfactory bulb, which is connected with the lateral ventricle [of the brain] by a small canal in the olfactory tract ... The olfactory tract is very short, but broad and [its wall is] made of white substance, which arises in the olfactory bulb and extends back to be continued [into the brain] by the olfactory striae. It [i.e. the olfactory tract] contains a canal which connects the ventricle of the bulb with the lateral ventricle [of the brain] ... The striae pass backward ... to the hemispheres.'[17]

The preceding quotation proves that Galen's description of the olfactory structures was correct when checked against the anatomy of those animals which he had an opportunity to dissect, except that there is no indication of perforations of the bulb toward the nose.—It also must be pointed out that Galen did not confuse the substance of the

16 Galen did not specify whether he dissected the nasal organs of the ox, horse or other animals. The olfactory structures of the horse are smaller than those of the ox. Only a description of the anatomy of the olfactory organ of the horse will be presented, because a pertinent detailed description of the nasal area of the ox, which Galen possibly dissected, was not available.

17 Sisson and Grossman, pp. 807ff. and 860.

brain with its ventricles, as suggested by some recent publications[18]. In most instances, Galen's dissections were exceedingly accurate as can be confirmed by a study of the same material. Since he dissected only the brain of animals, we had to relate his anatomical description to veterinary treatises of the animal species indicated by him, such as horse, ox and ass.

Galen was thus convinced that the olfactory tract was not a true nerve but, like the brain, surrounded by meningeal membranes through which the true cranial and peripheral nerves had to pass to their peripheral destination. As mentioned before, the thin sensory fibers extending from the olfactory bulb to the nasal mucosa (p. 141 and Fig. 10) had escaped his attention. Because a specific peripheral olfactory nerve did not seem to exist, all odors had to rise from the nose to the olfactory bulb. We will better appreciate these ideas if we quote Galen's own treatise, where he distinguished the olfactory organ from the cranial nerves:

> 'Whoever desires to enumerate simply the processes arising from the brain will say that the first pair of nerves springing from the brain goes to the two nasal cavities, and its course travels along the middle region of the skull. The second pair is that of the optic nerves, and in their course its two components travel one on each side [alongside] the nerves of the first pair. The third pair is that of the nerves which move the eyes [oculomotor nerve]. Nevertheless, anyone who does not wish to reckon simply the [cerebral] processes but the nervous processes and their points of origin will count the optic nerves as the first pair, and as the second pair that of the nerves moving the eye.'[19]

A few pages later, Galen gave another brief summary of his identification and numeration of the cranial nerves. He again counted the olfactory organ as a part of the brain but the optic nerve (our second cranial nerve) as the first nerve (see also the chapter on cranial nerves on p. 6).

18 Kollesch, p. 109, note 2, referring to Leyacker (1927).
19 Duckworth, p. 188; Simon, vol. 2, p. 172.

B. EXCRETION OF RESIDUES THROUGH THE OLFACTORY ORGAN

In *De usu partium* [12], in a special treatise *The olfactory organ* [20], and in some chapters of the *Anatomical procedures* which have come to us only in the Arabic translation (Duckworth, Simon), Galen not only described the olfactory bulb and tract as part of the brain in contrast to the true cranial nerves, but also as an excretory organ:

> 'There are two excrescences of the brain, long and hollow, which extend downwards from the anterior ventricles of the brain to those parts of the skull where the nose begins. This is the location of the ethmoidal bones (*ethmos*, sieve) the name of which explains their function. Here, the dura mater is perforated by fine openings where it touches the cranial bones [lamina cribrosa]. Also the heavier waste products [of the brain] are filtered through these holes. Since the time of Aristotle, it has been customary to call these waste products *perittomata* . . . Thus, the heavy discharges, called *blenna* and *coryza*, are secreted downwards . . . into the channels of the nose [located between the turbinate processes and the roof of the nose] . . . the thicker discharge flows into the mouth through the openings already mentioned . . . and these are covered with a bloodless membrane which spreads to the ethmoids while others are evacuated from the nasal openings.' [21]

But Galen explained that the olfactory tracts drained not only the lateral ventricles of the brain, since an additional drainage was furnished through the spongy ethmoid bone to the posterior nasal cavity and the pharynx (see Fig. 4 where the infundibulum points toward the ethmoid bone). Galen wrote:

> 'Both anterior ventricles have a narrow and long outgrowth [literally termination, *teleuten*] at the anterior, lower end, where the nasal canal enters [the brain] (i.e. the olfactory tract). However the upper opening [of each lateral ventricle] turns wider to the middle,

20 Kuehn, vol. 2, pp. 857–886 (translated by Kollesch, 1964).—Quotations from the other treatises are given in the text.
21 Kuehn, vol. 2, pp. 859–860 (condensed). See figure 4.

from here into an oblique canal and then down to the base of the brain [i.e. through the third ventricle into the infundibulum].'[22]

In other words, Galen described both an anterior drainage leading from the cerebral ventricles via the olfactory organ to the nose, and a posterior channel via the pituitary gland and the infundibulum (funnel) equally terminating in the nasal cavity. This doctrine is confirmed by Galen's treatise *De usu partium*[23] where he described this arrangement as a protection against the retention of mucus in the brain and thus as a safeguard against strokes. Evidently, Galen did not regard the nasal secretion *(phlegm)* as a product of the mucosal lining of the nasal cavity itself as we do today, but as an excretion of the cerebral ventricles. Since the air-channels leading to the cerebral ventricles likewise passed through the olfactory organ, the brain was in this manner also protected by a filter mechanism against inhalation of toxic fumes and noxious odors.

C. INCONSISTENCIES OF GALEN'S DOCTRINE OF SMELL

Three difficulties arose, however, from Galen's olfactory doctrine. One concerned the respiration of the brain. As explained elsewhere[24], Galen had postulated that the quality of heat, carried by the inhaled air, was absorbed in the lungs, transformed in the pulmonary blood vessels and in the left heart into vital pneuma, and carried by the arterial blood through the whole body. The vital pneuma was further transformed into cerebral pneuma in the vascular coils of the carotid arteries, i.e. the *rete mirabilis* and the *choroid plexus*, both located close to the base of the brain[24]. An exception from this rule was, however, the assumption that for perception of odor the air should flow completely unchanged from the nose into the anterior cerebral ventricles. This outside air was thought to be transformed in the cavities of the brain directly into *cerebral pneuma (spiritus animalis)* without participation of the abovementioned blood vessels. With air, Galen reasoned, the odoriferous particles could enter unchanged directly into the ventricle of the olfactory bulb (p. 142).

22 Kuehn, vol. 5, p. 613; see fig. 4, p. 63; also Siegel, fig. 7, p. 119 (1968).
23 Kuehn, vol. 3, p. 651; Galen, *De usu partium*, book 8, chap. 7.
24 Siegel, p. 154, 113 (1968).

The second contradiction resulting from Galen's olfactory doctrine was that the olfactory stimulus was supposedly perceived immediately by the brain, whereas all other sensory stimuli had first to be taken up by a peripheral sense organ before they were conducted by a specific nerve to the brain. It did not occur to Galen that such inconsistencies weakened rather than supported his physiological doctrines of perception. However, Galen was more inclined to accept contradictions than to abandon some traditional doctrines [25]. This tendency was greatly strengthened by his inclination to derive functional concepts from anatomical observations. In this particular instance, the mistaken anatomical demonstration of nasal pores seemed to lead to the erroneous ideas about olfactory perception and the entrance of unmodified air into the cerebral ventricles.

Thirdly, it seems strange that Galen believed in a two-way passage through the openings between the nose and the olfactory organ, upward for odors, downward for mucous residue. However, the loose structure of the ethmoid bone appeared to permit that two apparently conflicting functions could take place in the same location. It has been already discussed that Galen spoke frequently of a two-way passage through other biological channels, since this concept was strongly supported by HIPPOCRATES [26], who mentioned a two-way flow of air in the trachea, the alternating swallowing and vomiting through the esophagus and a two-way passage through the vaginal canal during fertilization and birth.

The doctrine of cerebral drainage through the olfactory organ persisted as a dogma and was accepted by all physicians until, in 1672, RICHARD LOWER was able to prove experimentally and by painstaking observation that the nasal discharge was a local product of the blood serum, and that the hypothetical channels in the olfactory organ and the infundibulum did not serve to drain the ventricles. LOWER stressed that it was still an obscure and mysterious matter to most physicians how the 'catarrh' could flow in such a torrent as almost to suffocate a living creature [27].

For these reasons, Galen concluded that the olfactory perception was principally different from the other types of sense perception. The ventricles of the olfactory organ had to perform three functions: the

25 SIEGEL, p. 104ff. (1968).
26 SIEGEL, p. 245 (1968).
27 LOWER, edited by HUNTER and MACALPINE (1963).

receptive action of a peripheral nerve or sense organ; the conscious cerebral act of the perception of odors; and thirdly, an excretory function for the discharge of mucus. In all other instances the stimulating event was confined to a peripheral sense organ and transmitted by a nerve to the brain and its ventricles as seat of conscious perception.

Although Galen localized all perception into the ventricles or the substance of the brain without attributing specific functions to circumscript areas, he had described the olfactory system as a little brain in its own right, in spite of the open communication between the small olfactory ventricles and the large ventricles of the brain. Galen even indicated that the specific impression of odors was confined to the olfactory area. But he did not consider other parts of the brain as equally specialized for the reception of stimuli from the other sense organs[28]. In any event, Galen's account of the olfactory structures was the first approach to a localization of function in a circumscript area of the brain. But he also thought that the anterior ventricles participate in the awareness of odors.

D. RELATION BETWEEN PULSATION OF THE BRAIN AND PERCEPTION OF ODORS

Galen explicitly explained that the passage of odors through the pores of membranes and bone separating the nose from the olfactory bulb did not depend only on the flow of air through the nasal passages, concurrent with the respiratory movement of the thorax. Even direct installation of odoriferous substances into the nostrils had frequently failed to lead to perception of odor. Therefore, he considered that the olfactory organ, located deeply in the skull, attracted air and odors by suction. Expansion and contraction of the olfactory bulb appeared indispensable for the flow of odoriferous substances from the nasal cavity to the olfactory bulb. But mainly the spontaneous pulsations of the brain were considered to enhance this effect[29], since it evidently pulsated in the same rhythm (*kinesis*, literally motion), alternatingly attracting air and expelling cerebral waste products[30].

28 SIEGEL, p. 114 (1968).
29 KUEHN, vol. 2, p. 867ff.
30 SIEGEL, p. 45ff., 123, 193 (1968).

Galen did not compare the action of the pulsating brain to the heart beat. He described that the contraction of the different layers of the heart muscle successively constricted and distended the cardiac ventricles, ceaselessly attracting or expelling the blood[30], but that the bulk of the heart muscle itself seemed not to change during systole and diastole while its motion contributed to the flow of blood. In contrast to the action of the heart, the brain was contracting and expanding its volume without participation of muscles.

Although both brain and heart seemed to move spontaneously, Galen considered an entirely different mechanism responsible for the contractions of each organ. He spoke of 'compression of the brain' *(piloumenon)*, a technical term used for the compression of wool into felt; but he never employed this word to describe the contraction of the heart muscle. He stated that the spontaneous 'compression' of the brain did not even interfere with its stimulating action on the skeletal muscle. He assumed that the constriction of the volume of the brain-matter ('contraction') automatically attracted the air from the nasal passages[29], according to the physical law of the *horror vacui*. Galen wrote:

> 'It follows from the law of continuity that during contraction of the brain the outside air has to be inhaled as it has to be exhaled during expansion of the brain.'[31]

It is difficult for us to understand that Galen failed to recognize that the pulsation of the brain was synchronous with heart and pulse, especially since he often had the opportunity to observe the movements of the brain and its membranes during operative removal of parts of the skull after head injury or trephining[32]. Galen apparently never compared the rate of pulsation of brain and arteries. He also stated that the pulsation of the brain did not depend upon the respiratory shift of blood during the movements of the thorax (SIEGEL, p. 96, 1968).

31 KUEHN, vol. 2, p. 868; KOLLESCH, pp. 44–45. For the contractility of the heart, see SIEGEL, pp. 30–47 (1968).

32 Galen's remark that ARISTOTLE mentioned that some animals have a 'cover' of the nasal passages, which has to open before odor can be perceived, seems to apply to the trunk of the elephant, but has no bearing on our problems (KUEHN, vol. 2, p. 871). It does not appear likely that he was thinking that the mucosal folds in the nasal cavity acted as valves.

E. NATURE AND DIAGNOSTIC ROLE OF ODORS

The fact that Galen spoke of odoriferous particles needs some explanation. Galen considered the air as undivided matter, since he did not accept the corpuscular doctrine of the atomists. Occasionally, however, he contradicted this statement when he employed an atomistic terminology. Quoting PLATO, he wrote that we cannot perceive odors when the nose is covered by a sponge which absorbs the odoriferous 'particles' *(meros)* of the air [33]. Galen further stated that particles which exceeded the size of the pores could not pass through the *lamina cribrosa*. Furthermore, particles mediating visual perception, he wrote, must be much smaller than those causing acoustic sensation, and these again smaller than the odoriferous corpuscles [34].

We encounter such contradictions in the treatises of many authors of antiquity, since neither the atomistic nor the opposite view could explain all observed phenomena. Even ARISTOTLE, although he consistently opposed the atomistic view, spoke often of particles and units. It, therefore, appears unwarranted to classify the ancient scientists and philosophers too strictly into rigid categories instead of exposing the difficulties with which they consciously struggled.—It is also possible that occasionally Galen's treatises were altered by copyists or during transcription of his public lectures by educated slaves who used shorthand.

Generally Galen expressed his accord with the Aristotelian doctrine of odors, assuming that the specific smell is the result of a combination of air with a quality particular to the odor-emitting substance. ARISTOTLE wrote that he could not identify the carrier of the odoriferous qualities which can join either water or air, since we find perception of odors even in aquatic animals:

> 'The medium in the case of sound is air; but in the case of smell it has no name. For air and water have certainly a common characteristic which is present in both of them, and bears the same relation to that which emits smell as the transparent has to color.' (*On the soul*, 419 a 32 Loeb. Class. Libr., p. 109.)

33 PLATO, *Timaeus*, 66.

34 KUEHN, vol. 3, pp. 647–648; Galen, *De usu partium*, book 8, chap. 6; DAREMBERG, vol. 1, p. 547.

In most instances Galen remained in the frame of this general doctrine indicating that odors did not consist of atomic or corpuscular particles but represented the substance and qualities of the odoriferous body [35]. He stated that odors arise from practically all substances as invisible vapor *(atmodes)* mixed with the air (*to periechonti*, literally: that what surrounds) [36]. They appeared sufficiently delicate to penetrate through pores of the ethmoid bone into the olfactory ventricles where they produced the sensory stimuli *(ten aisthesin)* [36].

Galen said that it was difficult to find appropriate terms to describe the different odors, although he used such expressions as sharp, penetrating, strong, harsh and many others for the perception of taste. The best way of classifying odors seemed to him to divide all sensations of the olfactory organ into agreeable and disagreeable. Vapors of many drugs appeared to act by entering the body via the same paths as odors. Galen wrote that irritating substances caused headaches by directly affecting the cerebral ventricles. But he believed that a certain benefit was derived from inhalation or nasal installation of drugs such as pulverized black cumin. When the vapor of this drug reached the deepest recesses of the olfactory organ, it seemed to cause initially a severe headache, but ultimately to force the discharge of apparently superfluous matter from the nasal cavities by violent sneezing [37].

Galen declared that abnormal humors created offending odors which offer us pathognomic signs of certain diseases *(nosode semeia)* [38]. He greatly stressed the diagnostic importance of the abnormal odors emitted by diseased organs. Thus, he quoted in his *Commentary to Hippocrates' treatise 'On the humors'*:

> 'In some people the odors of the entire body and mouth are offending ... often due to neglect ... Others have putrid ulcers, decayed teeth, stomach ailments and other diseases.' [39]

35 KUEHN, vol. 2, pp. 864 and 884; KOLLESCH, pp. 42 and 62, referring to *ousia* and *poiotes*.

36 KUEHN, vol. 16, p. 214. See also p. 144. For characterization of odors: KUEHN, vol. 11, p. 698.

37 KUEHN, vol. 2, pp. 859, 866, 883; vol. 5, p. 628; see also SIEGEL, p. 320 (1968). These drugs were called *sternutatoria*.

38 KUEHN, vol. 1, p. 362.

39 KUEHN, vol. 16, p. 215.

He advised looking for the cause of bad odors by inspection of urine, stools, ears and sputum. Again quoting HIPPOCRATES, he wrote:

> 'One should arrange the observed symptoms according to categories . . . and search for the different sources in the qualities of these odors.'[40]

One should, however, pay special attention to the nasal discharges which constitute the evacuation of a diseased brain[41].

Galen took greater interest in describing various odors which exude from patients than in diagnosing the signs of a disturbed olfactory perception, although he mentioned in several treatises a disturbed sensation of smell. Such lesions of olfactory perception, he wrote, could occur by obstruction of the nasal passages; further, by blockage of the pores leading through the ethmoidal bone; and thirdly, by a disease of the anterior (lateral) ventricles of the brain[42]. Galen did not discuss any further details of these lesions but stated that odors were often apparent only to the patient without being noticeable to others. He also analysed olfactory hallucinations at great length, pointing out that such symptoms revealed little about the constitution of the patient, but that they constituted signs of imminent disease[43]. Since Galen was greatly interested in visual and auditory hallucinations, these questions shall be discussed in the special chapter in a later study of Galen's psychiatry[44].

40 KUEHN, vol. 16, p. 216.
41 KUEHN, vol. 16, p. 217.
42 Galen, *De locis affectis*, book 3, chap. 15; KUEHN, vol. 8, p. 214.
43 KUEHN, vol. 1, p. 362; in Galen's treatise '*De arte medica*', XXI.
44 In preparation.

IV. ORGAN AND PERCEPTION OF TASTE

A. TRANSMISSION OF TASTE

Galen wrote that the safest way to identify drugs is by tasting:

> 'Taste differentiates most [pecularities of drugs], whereas the sense of smell confirms poorly, as one says.' [1]
>
> 'There is a great similarity between perception of odors and taste.' [2]
>
> 'But it is common to all odors that they do not indicate, with any degree of safety, the mixture [of their basic constituents].' [3]

Galen thought that the sense of taste was more reliable than smell because odoriferous substances often secreted insufficient vapor into the air to stimulate the olfactory organ, whereas the tongue was directly stimulated by the elementary particles *(moria)* [4]. It should again be noted that this was an obvious contradiction to his usual anti-atomistic attitude. In the chapter on perception of smell it has already been mentioned that Galen occasionally considered very fine *(leptomesteroi)* particles in the inhaled air as the cause of odor (p. 155). Likewise, he suggested that the organ of taste was stimulated by yet coarser corpuscles [5].

Evidently Galen did not adopt ARISTOTLE's non-corpuscular concept of taste perception, that taste was mediated by the transfer of qualities from the object to the tongue. ARISTOTLE's concept was derived from the observation that water passing through other substances became 'charged' with certain qualities *(poion ti to hygron paraskeuazei)* which communicated the sensation of flavors [6].

1 KUEHN, vol. 11, p. 703.
2 KUEHN, vol. 11, p. 697.
3 KUEHN, vol. 11, p. 700.
4 KUEHN, vol. 11, p. 702; *ta moria ton geuston somaton prospiptei te glotte kai kinei ten aisthesin.*
5 KUEHN, vol. 7, p. 122.
6 ARISTOTLE, *De sensu*, 441 b 17.

The rapid advancement of anatomical knowledge made other aspects of ARISTOTLE's explanation of taste perception obsolete. ARISTOTLE had still insisted that the sensation was carried from the tongue by the blood to the heart, the common seat of all sense perception [7], [8] *(panton ton aistheterion koinon aistheterion he kardia)*. Arguing against the alleged error that the brain was the seat of sensation, ARISTOTLE had followed the concepts of PLATO [9] and earlier philosophers that the liver or the heart were the seat of the soul. They had disregarded that this concept contradicted their own idea of blood flow, since the blood was supposed to flow from the heart to the peripheral organs [10]. However, these conceptual difficulties did not interfer with Galen's study of the anatomical basis of taste perception. Galen had not only proved beyond doubt that the brain was the exclusive seat of all sense perceptions, but by detailed studies on the innervation of the tongue he was able to describe correctly the different functions of the three principal nerves supplying the tongue, and to demonstrate their origin at the base of the brain.

B. TRIPLE INNERVATION OF THE TONGUE

Galen determined the sensory or motor character of the nerves of the tongue by observing their degree of hardness. In most parts of the body the sensory nerves appeared softer than the motor nerves. It seems that Galen's results of differentiating two types of nerves according to their degree of hardness were fairly correct, although exceptions were not rare [11]. He thoroughly studied the functional loss after dissecting or crushing certain nerves in vivo in order to substantiate these observations.

7 ARISTOTLE, *On youth and old age*, 469 a 5–13.

8 The brain seemed to be more appropriate to receive the 'smoky vapors' connected with odor; but this argument did not seem to apply to taste (ARISTOTLE, *De sensu*, 438 b 26) and other sense-perceptions.

9 PLATO, *Timaeus*, 67 b 2ff. See also p. 25.

10 SIEGEL, p. 88 (1968).

11 Prof. CHARLES M. GOSS answered in a letter to my question about the hardness of nerves: 'The big sensory nerves, optic, acoustic, part of the trigeminal, are softer, but there are many smaller ones which have a firm consistency. The connective tissue-sheath of a nerve makes it hard, not so much whether it is a motor or not.' I want to thank Dr. Goss for this commentary. Galen even mentioned the common sheath of cranial nerves as a possible source of error (see p. 9), but mainly referred to the sensory or motor character of the peripheral nerves by relating their function to their respective origin from 'softer' or 'harder' areas of the brain.

Galen wrote that three different pairs of nerves supply the tongue: the lingual, glossopharyngeal and hypoglossal nerves (modern terms). The lingual was a part of the third branch of the third nerve (Galen's numeration), corresponding to the lingual branch of the 5th nerve of modern nomenclature (trigeminal nerve).Galen thought that the lingual nerve communicated gustatory sensations. We know that it responds mainly to tactile stimuli, but has also some fibers sensitive to taste. Galen may even have been aware that the lingual nerve carried both types of fibers, since he wrote that this nerve was not considered by all anatomists as purely gustatory [12].

Galen described that the second nerve supplying the tongue was a part of the 6th pair of cranial nerves. He considered the 6th as a single nerve, although it contained three separate nerves which we describe today as the 9th, 10th and 11th cranial nerves: the glossopharyngeal, vagus and accessory nerves. Galen noticed that these different nerves were very close together at their origin from the brain, surrounded by a common sheath during the first part of their downward course [13].

One strand of these fibers, corresponding to the 9th nerve of our terminology, was already known to Galen as the principal gustatory nerve of the tongue. We call it the glossopharyngeal nerve. Although Galen considered that this nerve supplied the tongue with gustatory fibers, he stated correctly that it also sent motor fibers to the pharynx [14]. He wrote:

> 'From it, on the way to the tongue, a small offshoot goes to the wall of the pharynx, i.e. its muscular wall.' [15]

Most of the glossopharyngeal nerve, he wrote, entered the root of the tongue. He further observed that this gustatory nerve formed a flat layer under the external layer (i.e. the mucosal lining) of the tongue without extending into the underlying muscle of the tongue. Although Galen described that the sensory nerves of the eye terminate in the retina and those of the ear in the helix like a flat network, he denied

12 Galen, *De nervorum dissectione*, chap. 5; KUEHN, vol. 2, p. 837.
13 DUCKWORTH, *Anatomy*, p. 197.
14 DUCKWORTH, p. 79; GOSS, p. 331 (1966); Galen, *De nerv. diss.*, chap. 10; KUEHN, vol. 2, p. 841.
15 KUEHN, vol. 2, p. 841.

any structural similarity between the nerve-endings in these sense organs and those in the tongue. He employed, however, in all three instances the same term for the spreading out of the sensory nerve (*platynesthai*, from *platys*, flat). He determined the sensory function of the nerve fibers supplying the tongue by testing their degree of hardness. These detailed experiments will be discussed in the next chapter.—Galen correctly did not relate the vagal and accessory part of his 6th nerve to the tongue.

By further dissection, he established beyond doubt that the 7th cranial nerve (Galen's numeration; the hypoglossal or 12th nerve of modern count) furnished most motor fibers of the tongue. He wrote that this nerve originated at the end of the brain, near the upper end of the spinal cord, and that only the movements of the tongue were abolished when it had been damaged[16].

C. DISSECTION OF TONGUE AND NECK; DISCOVERY OF THE RECURRENT NERVE; GALEN'S EXPERIMENTAL METHOD

Most of Galen's interesting and detailed writings about the dissection of neck and tongue can be found in that part of his descriptive treatise on anatomy which has reached us in an Arabic translation (English edition by DUCKWORTH) and of which about 60 pages deal with the dissection of mouth, pharynx, larynx and neck. In addition, the treatise *De usu partium* (preserved in Greek) comprised a large chapter on the same topic which was translated into French by DAREMBERG and into English by MAY. Galen described the course of the recurrent nerve to the larynx, but without repeating the technical details of his experimental work on the recurrent nerve which we find in the translation of the Arabic text. He also discussed the innervation of the tongue in great detail in these chapters.

We know that Galen frequently dissected the horse, the ox, and other large animals[17]. As previously mentioned, he would have preferred to examine only apes because of their likeness to the human

16 DAREMBERG, vol. 1, p. 595; Galen, *De usu partium*, book 9, chap. 13; KUEHN, vol. 3, p. 735.
17 DUCKWORTH, *Anatomy*, p. 2.

body. But inspection of larger animals allowed him to recognize more details. In spite of their even greater differences to the structures of the human body, he occasionally dissected pigs and goats. For the study of the structures of the neck, he even examined birds. Knowledge of the anatomy of the neck already appeared important to Galen for practical reasons (see p. 164). Although other anatomists still questioned the role of the larynx for the formation of the voice, Galen was able to solve this problem by demonstrating that disruption of the recurrent nerves of the animal always paralyzed the vocal cords with consecutive total loss of voice. We can hardly find a more fascinating chapter of experimental medicine than Galen's studies of the larynx, pharynx, tongue and adjacent vascular, muscular and neural structures of the neck. A critical analysis of Galen's description of the most minute anatomical details would necessitate a thorough comparison of human and animal anatomy.

Therefore, we shall confine ourselves to a brief discussion of Galen's discovery of the recurrent branch of the vagus nerve (the 6th nerve of Galen's count). He was able to separate this slender nerve from the other nerves which supply tongue and throat. Besides, these careful dissections of the cervical organs enriched also Galen's knowledge of the structure and function of the tongue, but without contributing to a better understanding of taste perception, i.e. without further clarifying the doctrine of taste.

In the pursuit of these dissections Galen discovered that on each side of the neck a slender branch of the vagus nerve, after its downward course with the large vessels of the neck, returned from the upper thoracic area to the muscles of the larynx and the vocal cords. Because of this upward course between the large vessels and the laryngeal organs he called it the 'recurrent nerve'. On further search, he found the same anatomical relations in many species of animals and he even raised the question whether the long neck of certain birds presented a similar course of recurrent nerve. For this purpose he investigated the long-necked crane and the still larger neck of the ostrich. He wrote:

> 'As I saw the neck of these animals to be very long, I thought that it would not be possible for a slender nerve which has its origin on the brain [the vagus nerve] that it should descend first as far as the thorax, and that from there a portion of it should return, which would have to traverse the whole length of the neck. But in that

> point there is in creation no slackness or remissness, as in fact there is none in any other instance . . .'[18]

Galen found in the neck of these birds the same anatomical features as in shortnecked animals: the right recurrent nerve runs around the subclavian artery, the left one around the aortic arch[19].

Galen induced a temporary damage of the recurrent nerve by pressure or removable ligature, but found that after release of the compression the voice of the animal recovered. Bilateral section of the recurrent nerves completely abolished the voice, whereas other functions of the throat, tongue and thorax remained intact[20]. However, if he severed or damaged the 7th nerve (Galen's count; now the *hypoglossal nerve*), only the movement of the tongue was abolished whereas the perception of taste remained intact. Also the movements of speech, swallowing and breathing could still be performed normally. He wrote:

> 'The nerves of the seventh pair are distributed to the muscles of the tongue. You can very easily constrict this nerve with a ligature, and it will then be shown that the tongue remains flaccid as though paralyzed and impotent.'
>
> 'Also, it is best and most expedient, if you intend that after relaxation of the ligature the animal should be able to perform its natural function with that organ, you should not sever the nerves... After you have injured the [hypoglossal] nerve, by whatever sort or kind of injury you like, and you have deprived the tongue of voluntary movement . . . you can now, if you wish, stitch up the incision . . . leave the animal until its consciousness returns and it recovers from the transient agony in which it was plunged at the time at which the incision was made into it. The animal when it is in this state may be assumed to be thirsty. In that case, you will see that it soon drinks when it sees water in a vessel from which it can drink. Then, when it swallows down the water which it is drinking, you will see how the larynx moves upwards in exactly the same way as it raised itself up when the animal was uninjured and in its natural condition. This is one of the proofs that the contrac-

18 Duckworth, p. 87.
19 Duckworth, p. 205.
20 Duckworth, p. 208–212.

tion of the tongue has no part to play in the movement of the larynx.'[21]

Thus, Galen had been able to demonstrate that the functions of the recurrent branch of the vagus nerve and of the hypoglossal nerve were clearly distinct, in spite of the almost common origin of both nerves at the brain. He wrote further on the same topic:

> 'And when you compress the [right and left hypoglossal] nerves with the fingers, or ligate them with a cord, or cut them through, or when bruising or crushing has been inflicted upon them, then you deprive the tongue of the animal of its voluntary activity. And similarly you deprive the muscles of the larynx of their activity when you injure the nerves which join the larynx and grow in it, especially the recurrent nerve. The nerve joins and connects with the larynx in exactly the same places as those where we said that it joins and connects with the larynx in the body of apes.'[22]

As mentioned before (p. 160) Galen had found that the glossopharyngeal nerve (the 9th cranial nerve of modern terminology) descends for a short distance along the carotid artery and jugular vein before it turns to the tongue which it supplies with sensory fibers (p. 162). Galen undertook also experiments with these nerves in order to study different types of normal and abnormal respiration. But since this chapter deals only with sense perception of the tongue, discussion of these questions has to be omitted.

Galen studied the anatomy of the neck not only to learn about the mechanism of respiration, of swallowing and about the formation of voice and of speech, but also for the benefit of surgeons, who already at this period performed thyroidectomy for large goiters. In his own treatises Galen mentioned two cases of removal of a goiter where the physician did not use a knife in order to avoid damage to the voice of the patient, but divided the tissues with his nails.

> 'Everybody found it strange that the voice was damaged, although larynx and trachea remained intact. But when I demonstrated to

21 Duckworth, pp. 103, 107 (slightly arranged).
22 Duckworth, p. 91. The nervus hypoglossus contains mainly motor fibers for the tongue. The vagus nerve mediates swallowing.

them the phonetic nerve [i.e. the recurrent nerve] their astonishment abated.'[23]

To exhaust all possibilities, Galen even ligated the main artery at the neck. He wanted to demonstrate that interruption of carotid blood flow failed indeed to interfere with the voice, although it eventually proved fatal[24].

Galen's studies of the structures of the neck prove to us that his technique of dissection was quite accomplished. He had trained himself to a point that he could lay bare, with a single stroke of the knife, the nerve of the tongue (the hypoglossal nerve) on the living animal. He wrote:

> 'On a few occasions I make mistakes, because the proceeding is in itself difficult, and gives trouble in connection with the discovery and the searching out [of the parts desired]. And since that is so, then if once, twice or thrice you too miss your objective in that, you must not despair, but hope that you succeed the next time. So do not shun making these experiments, and do not interrupt or abandon them. It is indeed shameful and disgraceful that everyone is accustomed to bring themselves to voyage across the great expanses of the sea for the sake of wealth, and thereby to endure very great hardships, but as regards the knowledge and the understanding of the nature of things, it is their custom not to undertake the repetition of the same task time after time, unless there is some money to be got by that.'[25]
>
> 'If I complete this work that I have started [on ape and man], as is my intention here, I want to dissect those animals also which crawl, fly and swim, and to describe what there is to see in them. I do that, as you know, with the animal placed in front of me, while I am looking at the things about which I am talking, especially when I am describing the method to be followed in their dissection.'[26]

23 Galen, *On the affected parts*, book 1, chap. 6; DAREMBERG, vol. 2, p. 498; KUEHN, vol. 8, p. 52 ff.

24 KUEHN, vol. 8, p. 54; DUCKWORTH, p. 106; SIEGEL, p. 105 (1968), explained that the vertebral arteries often maintained the life of the animal for a considerable time.

25 DUCKWORTH, *Anatomy*, p. 214.

26 DUCKWORTH, *Anatomy*, p. 108 (arranged).

Galen unquestionably dissected these parts of the human body since the anatomy of the neck seemed to him a science neglected by those who performed thyroid surgery and treated operatively laryngeal abscesses and angina Ludovici, a phlegmone of the floor of the mouth (modern term for a disease already frequently mentioned by HIPPOCRATES). It becomes even more evident that Galen dissected the neck of human subjects when we read his own treatise on anatomy:

> 'The larynx is constructed in the same way in the bodies of apes and man, a construction which is shared by other animals which have a voice [i.e. such as pig and others]. You must, then, dissect a dead man and an ape and other animals furnished with a voice which have, besides the voice, the vocal apparatus of the larynx.' [27]

D. TASTE AND HUMORS

Since the innervation of the tongue appeared perfectly symmetrical, Galen believed that the tongue grew together from two parts like all other sense organs which are in pairs [28]. The existence of a split tongue in snakes confirmed this idea. ARISTOTLE had already suggested that one derived more pleasure from a double sense organ, since twofold stimuli could reach the center of perception [29].

The tongue itself seemed to be an organ of pale and soft texture into which the muscles entered together with the blood vessels and nerves [30]. Galen also described the submandibular salivary glands which are located directly beneath the tongue. He even probed the salivary ducts. Therefore, their excretory canal should rightfully be called after Galen, but not after BARTHOLIN or WHARTON. Galen wrote:

> 'On both sides of this band [frenulum] you find the orifices of ducts called salivary [ducts of BARTHOLIN or WHARTON]. On the tongue of an ox a thick sound [probe] may be able to penetrate into any one of these orifices, but with the tongues of small animals the use

27 DUCKWORTH, p. 86.

28 KUEHN, vol. 3, p. 712ff.; also DAREMBERG, vol. 1, p. 584; Galen, *De usu partium*, book 9, chap. 8.

29 ARISTOTLE, *Parts of animals*, 660 b 10.

30 SIMON, vol. 2, p. 47, and note 182.

of a fine sound is required for that purpose. The origin of these ducts is near the root of the tongue, where the spongy flesh [glandular mass] attached to the tongue lies, since the origin of these ducts is from that part.' [31]

We can find indeed that in most domestic animals the sublingual salivary glands are multiple and that their ducts unite on either side into one large duct which leads into the oral cavity below the tongue, near the midline [32].

Galen observed correctly the structural difference between the lymph nodes and salivary glands. He considered the lymph nodes only as support of the blood vessels, since he had found these nodes located mainly on the bifurcation of middle sized blood vessels [33]. He also recognized that the salivary glands produced an external secretion, whereas the lymph nodes yielded no secretion:

'Should you previously have detected their first [foremost] ending, which lies externally at each side of the frenulum, then insert a long slender sound [probe], whether of wood or of bronze, follow the sound and trace its course until you reach the gland which I have mentioned to you. But should you wish to begin and approach it from the glandular tissue which I mentioned to you, and which lies on the tongue, then incise the gland tissue through its sheath which invests all its several lobes [fleshy parts], and observe the roots of these vessels which discharge the saliva. Their original source is that spongy flesh [gland] and they are in fact like numerous fine rootlets which unite with one another, and from these arise other rootlets larger than the foregoing.' [34] 'This vessel which is called the salivary outlet [duct of BARTHOLIN or WHARTON] possesses, as I have remarked, two large rootlets on each of the two sides [of the tongue]. You see also that to this spongy flesh which I have mentioned are joined and connected a vein and an artery together. This is something which you must memorize in relation to all spongy flesh [glandular tissue] which has been created for the generation of some fluid from which the animal derives some

31 DUCKWORTH, p. 60.
32 SISSON, pp. 407, 489 (4th edition, 1956).
33 SIEGEL, p. 228 (1968).
34 DUCKWORTH, p. 61.

use. For this is a matter which is common to it all. Again, the nature of this spongy flesh, set apart for generation of fluid, is other than for support of blood vessels where they branch.'[35]

Galen stated elsewhere that moisture (saliva) was essential for taste perception, since only a moist tongue could function normally. Except for a greatly increased number of anatomical details about the sensory nerves, the modern doctrine of taste perception does not give us more information about the mechanism of gustatory sensation than Galen's statement, that we only taste substances in a fluid state, because they come in closer contact with the tongue. In Galen's words, perception of taste depended upon the presence of watery humors[36]: 'The organ of taste is moist and like a sponge.' He was convinced that the moisture of the tongue was derived from the humors of the blood vessels by the salivary glands.

It is difficult to identify the seven qualities of taste which Galen indicated, since some of these terms referred to almost identical impressions. We also are not too familiar with the implications of many words used by him. He spoke of bitter *(pikros)*, sweet *(glykys)*, salty *(halykotes)* and sour *(oxys)*. These four qualities are the only true qualities of taste which modern physiology accepts. But Galen had another word for bitter *(austerotes)*, one for a stringent *(stryphnes)* and an expression which can be translated as bitter, piercing or acrid *(drimys)*[37]. We know today that taste is closely associated with smell, since the four basic sensations of taste are usually mixed with odors when the nasal passages are open. Galen mentioned that the true number of gustatory qualities remained debatable[38]. Evidently, the description of the different aspects of taste proved to be as difficult as that of odors (see p. 156).

E. TASTE, AND INSPECTION OF THE TONGUE IN DIAGNOSIS OF DISEASE

In his discussion of the importance of function and appearance of the tongue for the diagnosis of disease Galen frequently referred to the

35 Duckworth, p. 61 (partly condensed).
36 Kollesch, p. 40; Kuehn, vol. 2, p. 864.
37 Kuehn, vol. 11, p. 445.
38 Kuehn, vol. 11, p. 450.

writings of HIPPOCRATES who had said that change in the color of the tongue indicated imminent disease. By inspection of the tongue HIPPOCRATES had tried to surmise the humoral disturbance causing the disease, regardless of whether the humors affecting the tongue seemed to come through the blood vessels or from the stomach[39]. According to his doctrine the tongue was a sensitive indicator of the prevalent humor in the blood stream[40]. Galen also referred frequently to the observation of HIPPOCRATES that the color of the predominant humor could be recognized by inspection of the tongue. Thus, the yellow tongue observed in jaundice confirmed the concept that yellow bile prevailed. A dark tongue seemed to indicate an excess of the black bile; an abnormally reddish tongue was referred to congestion, but a pale tongue to an excess of whitish phlegm[41]. Usually the color of the tongue seemed to match that of the urine[42].

Galen mentioned repeatedly that the tongue appeared black in inflammatory fever of the uterus *(phlegmonainouse metre pyretoi)*. He related this to an increase of black or yellow bile, the assumed cause of many fevers[43], but also stated that dehydration was the most likely cause of the discoloration of the tongue. We should remember that in Galen's time septic infection of the womb was exceedingly common.

It is difficult for us to reconstruct most of the clinical pictures described by the physicians of antiquity because of our entirely different interpretation and classification of observations. We can, however, recognize that Galen spoke of dehydration, when he stated that a dry dark tongue appears frequently in gastric fever and meteorism *(pneumatouses tou chymou)*, but rarely in 'black-biliary disease of the spleen'. In other words: septicemia or gastro-intestinal fevers, which he could not differentiate from other acute infections such as of the gallbladder or appendix, rendered the tongue dry and dark. But chronic disease, manifested by abdominal congestion with splenomegaly[44], did not lead to such a severe state of hydration of the body and, therefore, left the tongue unchanged[45].

39 KUEHN, vol. 17 b, p. 277.
40 KUEHN, vol. 17 b, pp. 278–279.
41 KUEHN, vol. 17 a, p. 343.
42 KUEHN, vol. 17 b, p. 270.
43 KUEHN, vol. 17 b, p. 273. See also SIEGEL, p. 275 (1968).
44 SIEGEL, p. 273 (1968), (possibly by malaria, schistosomiasis, cirrhosis).
45 KUEHN, vol. 17 b, pp. 273–274.

When Galen mentioned that a dark (literally black) tongue was a sign of high fever[46], he failed to refer to dehydration by excessive sweating. Increased insensible perspiration during fever was hardly discussed in the ancient literature. But Galen indicated this state of dehydration by describing such cases as suffering from 'dryness of the arteries and veins and even of the entire body'[47]. He also knew that when fever led to delirium 'the tongue became very dry'[48]. He stated that delirium could also be expected when patients with abdominal pain and yellowish, liquid bowel movements became restless and when their tongues became very rough and dry[49]. Loss of the desire to drink indicated the severe damage of both 'the state of consciousness of the patients and the abdominal organ'[50].

It is rather difficult to arrive at a modern diagnosis from such scanty remarks from Galen's treatises. The ancient physicians were mostly not attempting to diagnose the cause and seat of disease but to observe the symptoms. This method allowed them not only to make a prognosis but also to recommend the best available dietary treatment and physical therapeutic measures[51].

Galen himself pointed out repeatedly that changes in the appearance of the tongue and alteration of the patient's sensation of taste facilitated the diagnosis of the humoral changes. Often an abnormal sensation of odors, perceptible only to the patient, announced an impending illness. Galen compared these symptoms to the visual and auditory hallucinations frequently preceding serious disease[52]. He blamed, of course, the presence of abnormal humors in the tongue for the disturbed taste perception, since a similar mechanism was made responsible for abnormal odors[53]. An only moderate reduction of the normal discrimination of taste resulting from a dryness of the tongue appeared to Galen as a less serious symptom[54].

46 Kuehn, vol. 8, p. 47.
47 Kuehn, vol. 15, p. 472.
48 Kuehn, vol. 17 a, p. 531.
49 Kuehn, vol. 15, p. 740.
50 Kuehn, vol. 17 a, p. 531.
51 Siegel, p. 213 (1964).
52 Kuehn, vol. 16, p. 224.
53 See p. 157.
54 Kuehn, vol. 5, p. 634.

In a treatise dealing with diagnosis *(De morborum differentiis liber)* [55], Galen mentioned the interesting observation of abnormal changes in the size of the tongue. After he stated initially that he noticed occasionally a shrinkage of the tongue, he referred to an abnormal enlargement of the tongue. Discussing two patients in whom the tongue had grown to an unnatural size, he wrote:

> 'There are diseases in which an organ kept its natural form, but had become abnormally large. This was combined with the lesion of its function ... Thus, the tongue could become too large to be able to fit into the oral cavity ... This enlargement reminds of priapism. Nichomachus of Smyrna was a patient whose entire body had grown unproportionally large, that he was hardly able to move himself ... In another case the tongue had grown without any pain, became very large, but did not look like edema or skirrhos or inflammation. The tongue did not give away under pressure [like watery edema] nor had it lost its feeling; it also was not painful but simply had become enormously large without showing any other abnormality. Likewise both testicles and breasts were enlarged ... And the glands of the neck [*choiras*, a term used for scrofulous enlargement of lymph nodes] produced no little discomfort in the activities of the patient, because they became abnormally large [the question arises whether this was a malignant or nodular goiter, or both]. Also the angles of the eyes *(kanthos)* became greatly increased in size in this syndrome. Such growth is called *egkanthis*.' [56]

We may ask whether this description referred to cases of acromegaly. We know that this disease, representing the sudden onset of abnormal growth, occurs in adult persons. It involves all extremities; tongue, nose and skin, of the eyelids and the margins of the orbits become hypertrophic. Therefore, Galen spoke of *egkanthis*, a term which usually denoted a small tumor in the angle of the eye, but which referred here probably to the enlargement of the soft tissue around the eyeball. The swelling of the glands of the neck could be interpreted as

55 KUEHN, vol. 6, pp. 836–880.
56 KUEHN, vol. 6, pp. 868–870; for *egkanthis*: CELSUS: 7, 7, 10; Galen, *De usu partium*, book 10, chap. 11.

metastasis of a causative malignant tumor or as a concomitant goiter, a question impossible to answer. Galen did not present sufficient clinical details in his treatise that we could deduce a definite diagnosis, and he did not relate the various clinical symptoms to an assumed humoral disturbance. There is, however, no other known form of gigantism which would cause enlargement of the tongue. Hypertrophy of the tongue is very rare except in cases of acromegaly and myxedema (deficiency of the thyroid gland). But although myxedema can induce an enlargement of the tongue, it never will result in an abnormal growth of the body. On the contrary, when myxedema occurs early in life, the development of the body is stunted. A description of myxedema could already be found in the writings of HIPPOCRATES, but without reference to changes of the thyroid gland. HIPPOCRATES stressed as the most impressing symptom of these cases the slowness and clumsiness of the body and mind [57].

It appears, therefore, as the most likely interpretation of the passage just quoted that Galen described the enlargement of the tongue in acromegaly. This case report, which represents one of the many informative descriptions of clinical syndromes, gives us an impression of Galen's astute clinical observation.

Galen also noticed neurological disturbances of the tongue. Thus, he described that in strokes affecting only one side of the patient the sense perception and motility of one half of the tongue could be maintained. This seemed to confirm his conclusions from anatomical studies about the sensory and motor innervation of the tongue. However, when the intellect of the patient appeared affected, he concluded that the lesion was located in the anterior part of the brain or in its anterior ventricle, since he related motor disturbance of the tongue to the posterior area of the brain [58].

Tremor of the tongue was observed in cases of mental disability, of high fever *(phrenitis)*, as a sympathetic disease during involvement of other organs, or simply because of a general weakness due to 'dry constitution' [59].

57 SIEGEL (1960).
58 DAREMBERG, vol. 2, p. 590; Galen, *On the affected parts*, book 4, chap. 3; KUEHN, vol. 8, p. 229.
59 KUEHN, vol. 16, pp. 555–556.

In conclusion: Galen's anatomical description of the innervation of the tongue and of the recurrent nerve was an outstanding example of anatomical research and medical writing. Disregarding the earlier results of Galen's anatomical studies, a modern textbook of physiology [60] stated that not earlier than 1834 PANIZZA was able to define the glosso-pharyngeal nerve as the gustatory nerve of the tongue, the lingual branch of the trigeminal nerve as the nerve of touch, and the hypoglossal nerve as its motor nerve. Thus ultimately Galen's discoveries were confirmed. Furthermore, Galen did not pronounce a specific doctrine of taste as he had done in the fields of vision, smell and hearing. But he did pay great attention to the inspection of the tongue and to disturbance of taste in disease.

60 LANDOIS-ROSEMANN, vol. 2, p. 860.

V. TACTILE SENSATIONS: TOUCH AND PAIN

A. DEFINITION OF TOUCH

The Greeks, especially Aristotle, related every type of sense perception to contact *(haphe)*. The customary translation of the term *haphe* as 'touch' leads, however, to an obvious misunderstanding. Galen wrote that the skin responded to tactile stimuli only if brought in direct contact (*haphe*, from *hapto*, to grasp, touch) with the object, whereas the sensation of taste required merely 'contact' through moisture on the tongue; further, he stressed that air was needed as medium for the transfer of sound, and a mixture of air with an odoriferous quality for the perception of smell. Evidently in all sense perceptions other than those of the skin, a neutral agent was thought to communicate the sensory stimulus through 'contact' with the sense organ. Therefore, a one-sided translation of the word *haphe* as 'touch' would obscure our understanding of the principle which Galen and Aristotle wanted to suggest: namely, that sense perception occurs either by direct or by indirect 'contact'. This chapter will be confined to a discussion of touch in the stricter sense, i.e. to the sensations mediated by the cutaneous nerves and by the nerves on the surface of the internal organs.

B. ARISTOTLE'S DOCTRINE OF TOUCH

Aristotle defined perception of contact by touch *(haphe)* as the most basic property of all living organisms without which they could not exist [1]. He wrote that tactile stimuli arose only from immediate contact with the object, since they had not to be transmitted by a medium from the object to the sense organ [2]. In fact, touch appeared as the only type of sensation responding to an object placed directly on the perceiving organ, whereas an object placed on the cornea could not be

1 Aristotle, *On the soul*, 413 b 5.

2 Aristotle, *Parts of animals*, 653 b 20ff.

seen. Tactile sensation seemed to result from a reaction of the flesh, *sarx*, or an analogous structure, or of the tissue of the skin. Since ARISTOTLE preferred to describe the 'flesh' *(sarx)* of the skin as sensitive, without making any further inquiry of its structure, it seems appropriate to translate the word *sarx*, as used by ARISTOTLE, as '*sensory tissue*'. In short, perception of touch appeared to him as a universal and basic reaction not only of the skin but of all living matter[3].

ARISTOTLE thought that wave-like undulations of the blood conducted the sensory impressions from the skin to the heart; but he neglected to search for the anatomical basis of sense perception in the skin itself, since studies on peripheral nerves were almost unknown[4]. Physicians did not even distinguish clearly the nerves from the tendons.

ARISTOTLE did not relate the perception of touch to the presence of one of the four elements in the skin, since he stated that the tactile sense responds to a great variety of stimuli[5]. Although he noticed that tactile perception communicated a variety of impressions[6], he assumed that the peripheral organ of touch consisted primarily of the cool element, earth. It further appeared likely that touch, like taste, was to be perceived peripherally by an element contrary to heat, since the heat of the body seemed to be concentrated in the heart, the central organ of perception. ARISTOTLE rated the heart as the hottest region of the body, harboring the vital fire, while the cool elements, earth and water, prevailed peripherally (see p. 3, 4, introduction). Let us not forget, that ARISTOTLE still believed that the blood was the carrier of the soul and hottest in the heart itself.

C. GALEN'S DOCTRINE OF TOUCH

Although Galen had recognized the brain as the only seat of perception and mental activities, his doctrine of tactile sensation remained otherwise in accord with the traditional, mainly with the Aristotelian concepts of qualities, elements and humors. However, Galen's anatomical studies of the peripheral nerves advanced his understanding of sense perception far beyond the knowledge of his predecessors.

3 ARISTOTLE, *On the soul*, 422 b 19ff.; also ref. 1; see also irritability.
4 DETAILS see BEARE, pp. 180–201; ARISTOTLE, *On dreams*, 461 a, Loeb ed., p. 361 ff.
5 ARISTOTLE, *On the soul*, 435 b 4; 422 b 27.
6 ARISTOTLE, *Parts of animals*, 647 a 15ff.

Galen did not believe that separate parts (i.e. fibers) of the peripheral nerves were receptive to different qualities of tactile stimuli, since each peripheral nerve seemed always to react as a whole. He called this response *antibasis* which literally means resistance[7]. Although the skin evidently transmitted different types of information about an object, such as of its consistency, temperature and other qualities, the receptive organs such as the hand were, however, thought to be supplied by only one type of nerve. In contrast to the strictly sensory nerves (optic, acoustic), most peripheral nerves seemed even to carry both motor and sensory fibers[8]. Galen stated: 'All motor nerves serve also for sensory perception.'[9] He did not believe that motor or sensory messages were carried by different fibers and that some peripheral nerves reacted in a specialized manner to tactile sensations.

Although, as we know today, the cutaneous nerves carry subspecialized fibers for perception of touch and temperature and probably even for pain (see p. 191), about 80% of the cutaneous nerves are composed of only one type of fiber susceptible to the different qualities of cutaneous sensation[10]. Galen based his concept about the unity of the peripheral sensory nerve not on experiment but on the observation of mechanical injuries of the whole nerve. The refined testing of the separate nerve endings in the skin is, however, a modern technique. Galen's idea was correct in the frame of the anatomical knowledge of his time, but should not be considered as an anticipation of later concepts about sense perception. Describing the hand as an organ equipped for perception of all tactile qualities Galen wrote:

> 'There was no use for one organ of apprehension, for another for touch, for holding, for lifting and transferring things, and another for discriminating warm, cold, hard, soft and other distinguishing qualities of an object. However, by grasping, the hand can judge the nature of all these [impressions] together.'[8]

Galen stated that the stimuli received by the skin or the tissues lying beneath the skin were forwarded through the peripheral nerves

7 KUEHN, vol. 5, p. 634.
8 KUEHN, vol. 3, p. 109; DAREMBERG, vol. 1, p. 181; Galen, *De usu partium*, lib. 2, chap. 6.
9 KUEHN, vol. 5, p. 622.
10 HENSEL, p. 118.

to the brain. Although he distinguished tactile qualities such as dry, moist, cold, warm, soft, hard and others, Galen classified the perception by touch mainly according to psychological principles. Thus, he understood that sensations of touch and temperature were subject to immediate recognition, whereas the perception of qualities such as dry and moist, or of size and motion seemed to require a conscious judgement (*logismos*, also *episkepasthai*) [11]. This presented an anticipation of the concept that immediate perception by specialized nerve-endings has to be distinguished from the evaluation of complex impressions.

D. PERIPHERAL AND VISCERAL SENSORY NERVES

As stated above, Galen was convinced that each peripheral nerve served both motor and sensory functions, since the larger nerves such as the sciatic nerve seemed to respond equally to both motor and sensory stimulation [12]. He did not know that the motor and sensory fibers leave the spinal cord by separate roots before combining into a single peripheral nerve.

In extensive experiments, Galen had found that a transection of the spinal cord between different vertebrae of the cervical and upper dorsal spine interrupted sensory and motor function in hands, arms or legs, according to the level at which the experiment was performed [13]. Since he had failed to observe the short but distinct sensory and motor roots, these experiments convinced him that both functions were conducted by the same neural structures and could be abolished together. The posterior sensory and anterior motor roots of the spinal nerves were not discovered for another 1600 years (MAGENDIE, 1822).

Galen wrote, however, that purely motor and sensory nerves were clearly distinguishable by a different degree of hardness. He thought that this dissimilarity resulted from their origin in different parts of the central nervous system. Since the predominantly sensory cranial nerves came from softer parts of the brain, they also were softer than the motor nerves which originated in the harder spinal cord. Galen thought that

11 KUEHN, vol. 1, p. 598.
12 DUCKWORTH, p. 263.
13 DUCKWORTH, pp. 20–25.

some nerves were of intermediate hardness, when they exhibited a mixed function. He also noticed that some sensory nerves appeared harder when they were surrounded by a tougher membrane [14]. It was impossible for me to verify these statements, since Galen dissected mainly domestic animals. Generally, however, he came to a fairly accurate evaluation of the function of the peripheral nerves, although he obviously often used for evaluating nerve function other criteria than the degree of hardness or softness (see also p. 159).

When Galen stated that most peripheral nerves could serve both motor and sensory function, he did not consider the fibrous structure of these nerves. He had failed to realize that all spinal peripheral nerves were composed of fibers, although he had observed that the optic nerve formed the fibers of the retina. Therefore, he overlooked that motor and sensory stimuli were indeed conducted by separate parts of one nerve. In order to explain that injury of peripheral nerves often interrupted only the motor function while sensation was maintained, he assumed that the sensory reaction of the nerve required less energy *(dynamis)* than the motor response [15].

Besides the peripheral sensory and motor nerves Galen distinguished a third type of nerve as receptor of impressions from the internal organs [16]. He described that the vagus nerve, during its passage through the thorax, gives up a sensory branch which enters the pericardium near the coronary artery and sends a small side branch to the heart muscle itself [17]. Galen further described that the vagus nerve descends through the diaphragm to the abdominal organs 'so that these parts could attain a high degree of sensibility' [18]. The observation that the vagus nerve surrounds the cardia (i.e. the upper entrance into the stomach) with numerous fibers appeared to him of greatest interest, since it seemed to explain the frequently observed abnormal sensation and the often intense pain perceived in the epigastric area. Practically in all these cases Galen diagnosed stomach disease, hardly considering

14 DUCKWORTH, p. 79; also KUEHN, vol. 2, p. 613; vol. 3, p. 724; DAREMBERG, vol. 1, p. 589; Galen, *De usu partium*, lib. 9, chap. 11; also KUEHN, vol. 3, p. 740; DAREMBERG, vol. 1, p. 597; Galen, *De usu partium*, lib. 9, chap. 14.

15 KUEHN, vol. 7, pp. 113–114.

16 KUEHN, vol. 3, pp. 378–379; Galen, *De usu partium*, lib. 5, chap. 9.

17 DUCKWORTH, pp. 203–204; SIEGEL, p. 44 (1968).

18 DUCKWORTH, p. 220. See also the chapters on heart disease and sympathy in SIEGEL, pp. 332–352 and 360ff. (1968).

that pain could also arise from the heart. Only on one occasion did he relate pain to an irritation of the pericardium [19].

Galen wrote that visceral sensations such as heaviness and pressure in the abdomen were likewise relayed by the vagus nerve to the brain. More than all other sensations, severe abdominal pain seemed to lead to syncope. Galen described *syncope* (collapse) as an indirect (sympathetic) effect of gastric disease on the heart, since he believed that irritation of the cardia of the stomach traveled through both humors and connecting vagal fibers to the heart, especially to the left ventricle. This sympathetic irritation seemed frequently to induce fainting and collapse by suppressing the production of the vital heat in the left chamber of the heart [19].

Although in his description of sympathetic disease Galen attributed most abnormal sensations in the epigastric area to disease of the stomach, he did not know that these sensations can originate in the heart muscle. The following is a quotation of Galen's anatomical observations on which he based his clinical concept of syncope. He described the course of the sensory stimulus through the vagus nerve after its provocation in the gastric area, mostly by abnormal humors such as black bile:

> 'After it has passed beyond the heart, this nerve [vagus] encircles the esophagus, places itself continuously alongside it, and is, as it were, bound up together with it. And when it has traveled further with it, it joins the mouth [oesophageal orifice] of the stomach and infiltrates it, so that this part attains such a high degree of nervous sensibility and of relationship with the components of the nervous system that it is pre-eminent above all the other bodily parts in this respect, and for this reason it possesses a surplus of sensitiveness. From this nerve, which reaches to the mouth of the stomach, small branches go also to the whole of the stomach, and thus the chief part of this nerve-pair, as I have described, remains on the stomach; but the rest, that part of it which is left over, blends itself with the nerve of which we have spoken already, that is, the one which traverses the thorax to the roots of the ribs [sympathetic trunk], and [unites] with one after another of those nerves which take their

19 KUEHN, vol. 3, p. 500; DAREMBERG, vol. 1, pp. 446–447; Galen, *De usu partium*, lib. 6, chap. 18; SIEGEL, pp. 160, 362 (1968). This publication gave a detailed discussion of Galen's concept of 'heart-disease', syncope and cardiac pain.

outflow from the lumbar vertebrae. Then it distributes itself to all the abdominal viscera, that is, the bodily organs in the abdomen below the diaphragm, and to the intestine.' [20]

It has to be pointed out that Galen did not recognize that the vagus nerve supplies also motor and secretory fibers to the stomach and other abdominal organs, since he considered these functions as completely independent of innervation and as a response only to local stimulation of the bowels. His interpretation of the vagus nerve as a purely sensory nerve was not based on experimentation but derived only from anatomical observation [21]. Although we are aware today that the vagus comprises some sensory fibers for visceral sensation, we still have no evidence that these fibers relate the perception of angina pectoris or cardialgia, i.e. stomach pain in the stricter sense of the ancient term [22]. We know, however, that the pain of angina pectoris is conducted from the diseased heart via the sympathetic fibers and the spinal cord to sensory centers of the brain. Galen, misjudging the sensitivity of the heart muscle, related syncope to a critical diminution of the combustion in the left ventricle.

As the last quotation illustrated, Galen already saw the numerous anastomoses between the abdominal branches of the vagus nerve and the sympathetic fibers visible in front of the spinal column [23]. Since the sympathetic nerves were very difficult to identify by inspection alone, he could not distinguish between the two functionally separate parts of the autonomous nervous system. In fact, it was extraordinary that he even noticed these sympathetic structures which, as we believe to-

20 Duckworth, p. 220.

21 Daremberg, vol. 1, p. 591; Galen, *De usu partium*, lib. 9, chap. 11.

22 Siegel, p. 344 (1968). See also next chapter, p. 187.

23 Duckworth, p. 221. For those not familiar with the anatomy of the visceral nervous system: the sensory fibers of the intercostal nerves originate, on each side of the spinal column, from the ganglia of the posterior roots of the spinal nerves. In the thorax an intercostal nerve runs along each rib.—The sympathetic fibers arise from the sympathetic ganglia which form a double chain alongside the anterior right and left borders of the entire spinal column. Each sympathetic ganglion has connections with those next to it. Sympathetic fibers extend also from these ganglia to the spinal cord and to all thoracic and abdominal viscera.—The vagus nerve arises in the pontine region, i.e. the lower posterior part of the brain, from where it descends along the carotid artery through the thorax to the abdomen, where it also forms some ganglia. The vagus gives up branches to all thoracical and abdominal organs. Thus, the viscera have a double innervation by both vagus and sympathetic fibers.

day, conduct most sensations from the abdominal or thoracical organs to the brain. Galen's concept of the vagus nerve as the only mediator of abdominal pain and syncope resulted evidently from the observation of the numerous anastomoses between vagus and sympathetic fibers. The role of sympathetic fibers in shock was yet unknown.

In the framework of his general doctrine of nerve action, Galen considered the awareness of hunger also as a 'tactile' stimulation of the gastric nerves by local humors [24]. He therefore believed that the regulation of food intake was likewise mediated by sensory vagus fibers of the stomach. We know today that the movements of the stomach, including the so-called hunger contractions, result from a central stimulation of the motor fibers of the vagus nerve, but we do not yet know the sensory mechanism which provokes the primary sensation of hunger. It even remains uncertain whether the vagus or another nerve communicates the feeling of hunger to the brain [25].

E. RECOGNITION OF TACTILE QUALITIES: THRESHOLD OF SENSATION

Like Aristotle [26], Galen believed that an ordinary, i.e. moderate stimulation of the sensory nerves in the skin resulted in tactile impressions such as touch or temperature, but that a violent irritation of these nerves provoked pain. Until recent times, the existence of separate pain receptors in the skin has still been questioned, since it appeared likely that only an exaggerated stimulation of the tactile receptors affected us as pain [27]. It is now, however, generally accepted that specific pain receptors in the skin do exist [28].

This chapter will be restricted to the discussion of Galen's concept about cutaneous sensations other than pain, since Galen's doctrine of pain perception is the topic of a later chapter. Galen thought that the

24 Kuehn, vol. 7, p. 130. Also Kuehn, vol. 3, p. 378.
25 Wright, p. 247ff.
26 Aristotle, *Parts of animals*, 648 b 15ff.
27 Landois-Rosemann, vol. 2, p. 864; Wright, pp. 57–63. Hensel referred to von Frey's theory (1914) that 'the central nervous summation of nociceptive (*nocere*, damage) stimulations can cause pain in absence of a specific pain-receptor'. Hensel, p. 213. See also chapter on pain, p. 184.
28 Hensel (p.213) referred to Achelis (1939) who spoke of specific pain receptors: see chapter on pain, p. 184.

impressions of touch, warm and cold were immediately perceptible, basic sensory qualities, whereas the recognition of other 'qualities' such as hard, soft, dry and moist required more than direct stimulation of the peripheral nerve[29]. Galen correctly considered these complicated tactile sensations as the result of a judgement *(logismos)* based on experience (p. 177). We know today that—except for pain—three basic qualities (touch, warm and cold) can be separately perceived by specialized cutaneous nerve-endings. All other tactile impressions appear to us as complicated psychological experiences, derived from the basic cutaneous sensations.

With reference to touch and temperature, Galen explained that tactile perception depended definitely on the condition of the receptive organ. He had noticed that not every contact elicited a sensation[30]. Thus, unless the amount of 'cold' of an object exceeded the amount of the same quality present in the stimulated area, a sensation of cold appeared impossible. Galen probably derived this idea from the writings of ARISTOTLE who had pointed out that sense perception depended on the state of the sense organ itself, but not on the absolute strength of a stimulus. ARISTOTLE assumed that an object must contain more of a certain quality than the skin if it is to be perceived. ARISTOTLE further believed that the qualities of an object could act upon the opposite qualities of the sense organ. He wrote:

> 'This is why we have no sensation of what is as hot, cold, hard or soft as we are, but only of what is more so, [i.e. of an excess] which implies that the sense [perception] is a sort of mean between the relevant sensible extremes [literally opposites]. That is how one can discern sensible objects. It is the mean that has the power of discernment; for it becomes different in relation to each of the extremes in turn; and in order that we better perceive white and black, it must be actually neither, but potentially both (and similarly [is it] with the other senses), as in the case of touch it must be neither hot nor cold.'[31]

29 KUEHN, vol. 1, p. 598. Galen's analysis was expressed in the quite difficult terms of humoral 'physiology'. An enumeration of 14 qualities was given (KUEHN, vol. 8, p. 692).

30 KUEHN, vol. 1, p. 563; vol. 3, p. 110.

31 ARISTOTLE, *On the soul*, 424 a 2ff. (p. 135, slightly modified).

If we want to state ARISTOTLE's idea in terms more familiar to us we could say that the intensity of each stimulus depended on the relative concentration of a certain chemical substance present in the sense organ. The 18th century physiologist H. WEBER expressed this idea adequately and briefly: 'We feel not a stimulus but differences between stimuli.' ARISTOTLE's and Galen's concept represented an anticipation of the modern idea of threshold of perception. However, we apply here a terminology entirely different from the humoral doctrine, which was the scientific language of Galen's time. The ancients judged temperature by the assumed quantity of hot or cold, whereas we associate with it a mechanistic concept of chemical transmittors.

Galen observed that severe cooling suppressed tactile sensation almost as completely as the mechanical interruption of the sensory nerves. The well known experience that cold relieves pain evidently supported this idea [32]. According to the general doctrine of qualities, the 'cold' seemed to lower the sensory response of the nerves by overpowering the other qualities.

Galen also described that another quality, besides the cold, was capable of suppressing all sensation. He referred to the startling observation that people suffered by contact with the electric torpedo fish a loss of sensation, even coma and stupor [33]. When such patients were rendered temporarily insensible, Galen spoke of *anaisthesia*. His impression was that an unknown quality emanating from the fish inactivated their nervous system by changing the balance of its constituent qualities. Often the shock inflicted by the torpedo fish left the sensation only partly disturbed, but completely abolished motion. Even passive movements of the extremities proved to be very painful [33]. Galen's interpretation of this phenomenon was likewise based on his concept of qualities in relation to the mechanism of nerve action [34]. A further consideration of Galen's ideas about pain will shed more light on his physiological ideas of tactile perception.

32 DAREMBERG, vol. 2, p. 506ff.; KUEHN, vol. 8, p. 70ff.; Galen, *De locis affectis*, lib. 2, chap. 2.

33 KUEHN, vol. 8, p. 72.

34 A detailed analysis of these problems has been given by SIEGEL, pp. 149, 177, 318 (1968); see also p. 47.

F. PAIN: PHYSIOLOGICAL AND PSYCHOLOGICAL CONSIDERATIONS

1. Humoral and Structural Causes of Pain

Galen considered pain as an important symptom from which he often attempted to deduce a correct diagnosis. He wrote:

> 'If we could check the cause of pain, we would not only be able to overcome the symptoms but really treat the illness itself. If, for some reason, we are unable to counteract the dyscrasia of the humors, at least we should be in a position to alleviate the intensity of the pain.' [35]

Galen's commentaries on pain were scattered among numerous treatises. Only his book *On the diseased parts* included some chapters in which he systematically analyzed the nature of pain[36].

Frequently Galen referred to the writings of earlier authors who had tried to determine, from the patients' complaints, the exact location of the disease. Thus, Galen discussed at great length the numerous references to pain which he found in the aphorisms and case histories of HIPPOCRATES.

Galen also devoted much critical thought to a treatise on pain by ARCHIGENES. He disagreed with this writer in many points, and rightly so, as this discussion will confirm. ARCHIGENES, a well known physician and greatly appreciated as a scientist, lived in Rome before Galen, at the time of the emperor TRAJAN (98–117 A.D.). Our knowledge of his medical writings derives mainly from Galen's references[37] who mentioned that ARCHIGENES wrote three important books on *The diseased parts (ton peponton topon)*. Galen evidently used the same title for his own treatise which dealt with diseases of internal organs.

Like his predecessor, Galen tried to deduce his diagnosis of a generalized humoral disturbance not only from the observed symptoms, but often from the complaints of pain, unmindful of whether or not he

35 KUEHN, vol. 10, p. 850; Galen, *Meth. medendi*, book 12, chap. 7.
36 KUEHN, vol. 8, pp. 69–119; DAREMBERG, vol. 2, pp. 506–533; Galen, *De locis affectis*, book 2, chap. 1–9.
37 METTLER, p. 506.

could find localized signs of disease. That Galen devoted special attention to the localization of pain is evident from the following quotations:

> 'In regard to the patient's symptoms, pain is either indicative of the diathesis [i.e. the composition of the humors] or it reveals the affected organ.'[38]
>
> 'The principle for [the recognition of] disease is the following: the function [of an organ] is never disturbed unless the part of the body, which produces this function, is affected; but if there is pain in a [certain] organ, this organ must definitely be diseased.'[39]

Always aiming at therapeutic measures and not only for the purpose of diagnosis, Galen classified painful symptoms into two groups: those indicating a diseased organ, and others expressing the assumed humoral disturbance:

> 'One has to distinguish between the proper signs of the diseased parts *(paschonton morion)*, and those indicating a disease [of the humors] *(ton pathon semeia)*.'[40]

Thus, Galen indicated that his concept of disease equally relied on consideration of humoral disturbances as on description of structural changes. Unfortunately, he often tried to support this view with inadequate examples. For instance, he considered indigestion *(apepsein)* as a symptom of a generalized humoral disturbance, whereas pain in the stomach impressed him as a sign of a strictly localized disease. More acceptable appears Galen's understanding of pleuritic pain:

> 'Evidently, if the pain affects parts of the body which have to move during respiration, it will render the respiratory movements shallow and frequent. In contrast, delirium *(paraphrosyne)* will cause deep and slow respirations. [Pleuritic pain could not be felt as long as a patient remained unconscious]. But when pain and delirium occur together, the relation between pain and respiration becomes confusing.'[41]

38 KUEHN, vol. 8, p. 70; DAREMBERG, vol. 2, p. 506.
39 KUEHN, vol. 8, p. 29; DAREMBERG, vol. 2, p. 483.
40 KUEHN, vol. 8, p. 43; DAREMBERG, vol. 2, p. 491. See also SIEGEL, p. 211 ff. (1968).
41 KUEHN, vol. 7, p. 849 (condensed).

Galen explained the pain of pleurisy as the result of a swelling of the intercostal arteries and muscles, since he knew that only the intercostal nerves conducted painful sensations from the surrounding structures to the central nervous system [42].

Referring to a chapter on abdominal pain in the Hippocratic treatises, Galen affirmed that small and frequent respiration usually indicated an affection of the diaphragm or of the organs below the diaphragm, i.e. liver, spleen, stomach, especially however of the cardia, which he defined as *stoma tes koilias*, 'the opening of the cavity'. He also recognized that lesions of the peritoneal covering of the lower surface of the diaphragm seemed to interfere with respiration [43]. Evidently, a topographical diagnosis of disease and its symptoms was Galen's goal.

Well aware of the difficulties of a detailed diagnosis, Galen indicated that pain on the right side of the abdomen usually resulted from disease of the liver or kidney, whereas pain on the left side suggested involvement of the liver, spleen or stomach [44]. Galen even mentioned injuries of the lower ribs or the diaphragm as worthwhile of consideration for the differential diagnosis of abdominal pain.

Galen was convinced that a localized disturbance of the humoral balance was a common cause of pain. This, he thought, could already be proved by the observation that pain could be suppressed by external application of cold. Galen understood that the analgesic effect of cooling resulted from a shift in the balance of humors (or qualities) in the painful area. Likewise he explained the numbness of the extremities after exposure to freezing temperatures as the effect of localized humoral changes, since he noticed that sudden warming of frozen extremities induced pain by transfer of the quality of heat. Failing to recognize the destruction of tissue by the frost bite, he attributed this pain to the effect of the opposing qualities of cold and heat on the tissue.

Galen often attributed pain to the influx of toxic black bile or acrid yellow bile [45] which probably by deterioration of blood and pneuma would lower the temperature of the body sufficiently to cause spasms at the upper opening of the stomach *(kardia)*, or induce paralysis *(parapleges)* of the limbs or even epileptic convulsions. He also believed

42 Duckworth, p. 218; Kuehn, vol. 8, p. 76; Daremberg, vol. 2, p. 510.
43 Kuehn, vol. 7, pp. 908–910; also vol. 18 b, p. 76. Siegel, p. 250 (1968).
44 Kuehn, vol. 18 a, pp. 13–15; Kuehn, vol. 11, p. 261; Kuehn, vol. 8, p. 45.
45 Kuehn, vol. 15, p. 779.

that humors other than black and yellow bile could equally provoke pain by changing the basic constituents in different parts of the body.

Thus Galen explained the pain of apparently ischemic or thrombotic areas of the body by surmising that the blood, when cooled by humoral changes, lost its usual fluidity and congealed. The vena cava and the other veins *(phlebes)* leading to the intestines seemed frequently affected. He related this condition to observations on dead bodies, where he mostly found clots in the veins whereas the arteries appeared empty [46]. Although Galen considered that the arteries carried blood, an inconsistency of terms was still prevailing. Evidently Galen referred to HIPPOCRATES who used the term *phlebes* for both veins and arteries, while Galen himself employed it only to indicate veins. Since we cannot know whether Galen noticed clot formation in diseased arteries we shall not decide whether the pain of these patients was due to ischemic disease of the extremities or to painful thrombosis of peripheral veins. Galen referred repeatedly to the 'obstruction' of blood vessels by the abnormally heavy and cool blood as cause of *paraplegia*, *apoplexia* and epilepsy [47], because HIPPOCRATES had attributed these diseases to clogging of blood vessels (phlebes), irrespective of pain. However, Galen considered that pain not only arises from damage inflicted by diseased humors to a single organ, but that the original disease frequently provoked pain in remote areas of the body by transfer of a morbid irritation.

2. *Sympathetic ('Referred') Pain*

Galen defined the communication of pain to other areas of the body as sympathy (*sympatheia*, suffering together). He attributed one type of sympathy to structural, mainly neural connections, another to a humoral transmission between distant organs. In both instances he distinguished the primarily affected organ as *protopatheia (protos*, first) or *idiopatheia* (*idios*, pertaining to) from sympathetically provoked pain in a second organ which he defined as *deuteropathia* (from *deuteros*, second) [48]. We would call the manifestations of such types of sympathy referred pain. It is remarkable that Galen thought that the communication of painful irritation through the nervous system does not indi-

46 KUEHN, vol. 15, p. 780.
47 KUEHN, vol. 15, pp. 775, 783; HIPPOCRATES' treatise *On diet in acute diseases.*
48 DAREMBERG, vol. 2, p. 494ff.; also SIEGEL, pp. 362–370 (1968).

cate a disease of the nerves itself. He even wrote that he never could find any visible changes in the peripheral nerves, even if all motor and sensory conduction became abolished. This remark strongly suggests that Galen dissected diseased and injured nerves of animals or patients [49].

Galen was exceedingly interested in the observation that sympathetic pain seemed to spread from the stomach to the heart, often with such an intensity that syncope (collapse) occurred. He wrote:

> 'You will find, when the stomach has become so hypersensitive, that severe symptoms can spread and transfer the damage to another organ.' [50]
>
> 'The heart can react by sympathy so violently to an affection of the stomach that acute collapse ensues.' [51]

Galen discussed whether the painful irritation would not spread directly from the stomach to the heart, but pass first via the visceral nerves to the brain and then descend to the 'sympathetically affected' organ, in this instance the heart [52].

Galen referred mainly to the sympathetic provocation of syncope (collapse, shock) but not to cardiac pain (p. 179). He was sure that a painful visceral irritation could be transferred by the vagus fibers, since by careful dissection he had discovered not only most ramifications of the vagus nerve but also sympathetic fibers (modern term) connecting the abdominal organs with the spinal cord. He even noticed the paravertebral sympathetic ganglia. In distinction to modern concepts, Galen did not differentiate the vagal from the sympathetic components of the combined visceral nervous system, but regarded the sympathetic fibers of the thoracical and abdominal organs as ramifications of the vagus nerve (the 6th cranial nerve of Galen's count). He interpreted the visceral system of vagal nerve as an alarm system which could be set in motion by noxious irritation [53], whereas 'normal' stimuli arising in the intestines seemed to remain unnoticed [54]. By speaking of the visceral

49 Kuehn, vol. 8, pp. 95–96; Daremberg, vol. 2, p. 521.

50 Kuehn, vol. 7, p. 136; see also this chapter p. 179, quotation No. 20 from Galen's anatomical treatise in regard to the vagus nerve.

51 Kuehn, vol. 8, pp. 341–342; Daremberg, vol. 2, p. 647.

52 Kuehn, vol. 7, pp. 137–139; for more details, see Siegel, p. 362 ff. (1968).

53 The so-called nociferous stimuli (modern term).

54 Daremberg, vol. 1, pp. 361–363; Galen, *De usu partium*, lib. 5, chap. 9.

nerves in similar terms as a 'third group of nerves' (p. 178), specialized for the perception of danger by sensing pain or distress[55], he anticipated the concept of the autonomous visceral nerves as a separate functional unit. Whether his teleological approach to visceral pain was justified remains a question which only can be answered according to one's personal philosophical outlook.

Galen thought that a certain constitutional predisposition raised the sensitivity of the intestinal nerves, when he wrote:

> 'Four conditions expose us to intense stomach pain by [producing a] hypersensitivity of this organ: the type of its nerves, the weakness of the arteries, of the cardia, or of the brain itself.'[56]

The same seemed to be true for the pain projected into or arising from the genital organs and the urinary tract.

Galen was only partly correct when he attributed the feeling of painful heaviness in the abdomen to an irritation of the sensitive nerves in the membranes (peritoneum) which not only seemed to cover the viscera but also to penetrate their tissues[57]. Extensive experimentation has finally established that only the parietal peritoneum (the layer covering the inner surface of the abdominal wall) is sensitive to pain, since it is supplied with sympathetic, sensory fibers originating in the spinal cord, whereas the membranes covering the viscera appear insensitive to cutting or pricking. Since in abdominal disease mostly both the visceral and parietal peritoneum are simultaneously affected, pain is usually transmitted through the connections with the spinal cord. Because of the difficulty in recognizing the detailed anatomical relationships, Galen wrongly attributed all visceral sensation exclusively to vagal connection, unaware that the innervation of the surface of the viscera by spinal sympathetic nerves was not of vagal origin.

55 *Lypesonton diagnosis*; KUEHN, vol. 3, p. 378; GALEN, *De usu partium*, lib. 5, chap. 9; DAREMBERG, vol. 1, p. 362.

56 KUEHN, vol. 7, p. 137.

57 KUEHN, vol. 8, p. 79; DAREMBERG, vol. 2, p. 511; Galen, *De locis affectis*, book 2, chap. 4; also KUEHN, vol. 3, pp. 309–310; Galen, *De usu partium*, book 4, chap. 13; DAREMBERG, vol. 1, p. 131; For modern anatomy: WHITE, J. C. (1955).

3. Subjective Varieties of Pain

Our understanding of the numerous subjective varieties of pain has not much advanced beyond Galen's account. We find that a modern textbook of physiology distinguished pricking, cutting, drilling, burning, lancinating, pulsating, pressing, gnawing and tearing pain, stating that the causes of these differences in quality remain completely unexplained[58]. Similarly Galen spoke of pulsating *(sphygmodes)*, heavy *(barys)*, sharp *(oxys)*, tension pain *(tonodes)*, punctuating *(nygmatodes)*, dull or numb *(narkodes)* pain, and of pain of ulcerating character *(helkodes)*. He further differentiated a periostal pain caused by inflammation of the membrane lining the bone, or pain resulting from external injury[59]. Galen mentioned that pain also could arise from an uncomfortable position during sleep, when the patient suddenly and quickly moved and stretched, twisting his cold and stiff limbs. Even the pain caused by sprains had a name *(tilma)* different from that occurring from muscular cramps *(spasmos)*[60].

Galen pointed out that it appears difficult to understand the various types of pain reported by another person and, since no adequate terms existed, even to describe the various personal impressions. He wrote:

> 'It is evidently impossible to transmit the impression of pain by teaching, since it is only known to those who have experienced it. Moreover, we are ignorant of each type of pain before we have felt it.'[61]

We find this idea expressed with almost the same words in a modern treatise on pain:

> 'Doctors who have been dealing with patient's pain for many years often express extreme surprise when they experience such visceral pain themselves. The diversity of painful experience must be almost unbelievable. Without experiencing it we can only guess at its variety and range.'[62]

58 LANDOIS-ROSEMANN, p. 874
59 KUEHN, vol. 8, p. 104; DAREMBERG, vol. 2, p. 525.
60 KUEHN, vol. 17 a, p. 763.
61 DAREMBERG, vol. 2, p. 532; KUEHN, vol. 8, p. 117.
62 KEELE, p. 155.

Pointing out that nobody could really know all possible types of pain unless from his own experience[63], Galen asked his listeners to arrange their studies systematically, first by describing clearly the different symptoms of pain, then by examining the changes in the affected parts and finally by searching for the cause of this affliction[64, 65].

4. *Specificity of Pain Sensation*

As explained in an earlier chapter (p. 178), Galen understood that pain was mediated by the mixed spinal motor and sensory nerves. He also did not assume a specific type of nerve as carrier of a painful sensation. Pain appeared to him merely as the effect of an abnormally intense stimulation of the sensory nerves, whereas moderate (physiological) stimulation seemed to evoke pleasurable impressions. Galen said that this rule applied to all, even to the specific nerves of ear and eye since extreme stimuli seemed always to cause a painful sensation in the acoustic or optic nerve:

> 'Pain is caused by unnatural and forceful stimulation (literally, affection) [of all our senses, *aisthesis*] as PLATO said, whereas mild (natural) stimulation appears agreeable [I read *epios*, not *apios*], since it corresponds to the character of the sense organ.'[66]

We know today that the sensory nerves of the eye or ear, which convey painful sensation after a strong illumination or a loud sound, are not part of the optic or acoustic nerve but are branches of the fifth (trigeminal) cranial nerve[67]. However, Galen did not yet distinguish the pain resulting from stimulation of these nerves from the pain provoked by excessive optical and acoustic stimulation. Therefore, we hardly can credit him with the anticipation of the correct understanding of the problem.

63 DAREMBERG, vol. 2, pp. 530–532.
64 KUEHN, vol. 8, p. 69; DAREMBERG, vol. 2, p, p. 506.
65 KUEHN, vol. 8, p. 43; DAREMBERG, vol. 2, p. 491; Galen, *De locis affectis*, lib. 1, chap. 4; see also quotations of ref. 39, 40.
66 KUEHN, vol. 7, p. 115.
67 WOOLLARD (1936); ref. in KEELE, p. 110.

Modern physiologists, well aware of the source of pain in the peripheral sensory organs, tried to find out whether cutaneous pain is perceived by fibers only receptive to painful sensation or the result of overstimulation of touch-receptors. In 1894 von FREY postulated that the stimulation of specific sensory points in the skin evoked the sensation of pain, but not of temperature or touch [68]. This doctrine was supported by STARLING [69], whereas almost at the same time GOLDSCHNEIDER advocated the idea that 'pain arises frequently from summation of stimuli which alone would not cause pain' [70]. It has recently been found that the pain-sensitive points have indeed not as much sensitivity to mechanical stimuli as those points which mediate other cutaneous sensations[71]. This discovery seems to explain Galen's impression that only an intense stimulus evokes pain in the skin, whereas mild irritation conveys the sensation of touch or even of pleasure. We have, however, to remain aware that Galen's intuitive deductions were methodically not comparable to the result of modern research. But even today the issue is still not settled (STERNBACH).

5. *Awareness of Pain*

Galen was aware that we cannot perceive pain unless the brain, the principal organ of sensation *(hegemonikon)*, was intact. He knew that suffering *(algedona)* depended on the normal participation of the brain and its ventricles. Absence of pain during evident irritation of the peripheral nerves appeared to Galen as a definite indication of mental disease [72]. He noticed that severe compression of the brain and consequently of the cerebral ventricles after injury or in animal experimentation caused insensibility (*anaesthesia*, loss of conscious perception for sensory stimuli). He called this condition *kataphora batheia* which literally means 'a deep sinking spell' (from *kataphero*, to bring down). Galen did not ask whether the pain was perceived only in a localized area of the brain, since he did not consider that different parts of the brain were endowed with a specialized function such as pain sensation

68 KEELE, p. 132.
69 STARLING, p. 434.
70 LANDOIS-ROSEMANN, p. 874; STERNBACH, p. 29–31 (1968).
71 WHITE, J. C., pp. 10–12 (1955).
72 KUEHN, vol. 17 b, p. 460.

(see discussion of localisation on p. 153). He believed, however, that the *cerebral pneuma (spiritus animalis)* served for separate functions in various parts of the ventricles of the brain, since experimental compression of the cerebral ventricles at different levels seemed to diminish step by step the state of consciousness [73].

Galen tried to distinguish between true and simulated pain 'by the criteria of medical experience'. He devoted a short treatise to the problem of 'How to detect malingerers' [74]:

> 'It is thus surely now clear that a combination of medical experience with the results of ordinary reasoning is useful in the diagnosis of extreme pain. From the fact also that the pain is well borne one may conclude that it is not very bad. This conclusion is often, of course, formed when people, who are pretending to be in great pain, unwittingly throw themselves about from one position to the other, although, forsooth, they pretend to be unable to endure their sufferings. Moreover, if they are really in great distress, they are prepared to put up with any remedy; in fact they are themselves the first to beg the doctor to do anything he chooses, so long as their trouble is cured. If, on the other hand, they are only slightly pained, or not at all, they flee from such remedies nor will they endure prolonged fasts or bitter medicines.' [75]

73 SIEGEL, p. 192ff., 306 (1968).
74 BROCK, pp. 225–228 (1929); KUEHN, vol. 19, pp. 1–7.
75 BROCK, p. 227 (1929); KUEHN, vol. 19, p. 6.

CONCLUDING REMARKS

With the advice of how to expose simulated pain (p. 193) Galen approached a discussion of the borderline between normal and psychopathic personalities. Since he devoted much thought to psychological problems, future studies would have to deal with the analysis of his concepts and observations in this field.

Earlier in this book it has been pointed out that Galen's studies on sense perception, especially on vision, have rarely been adequately appreciated. His studies, so rich in original observations and valuable suggestions, were hardly systematically pursued. This was already the case during the time of late antiquity and remained so during the Middle Ages and the Renaissance. To mention only one instance: Galen's detailed knowledge of the structures of the eye remained widely unknown; even VESALIUS published in the *Fabrica* an anatomical sketch of the eye which would have been already obsolete in Galen's time[1].

We can readily apply to our judgement on Galen and his successors KEILIN's advice: 'In looking back at the development of our knowledge we can see that it did not follow a straight or logical course. Not only do we learn much from past difficulties, but it often helps to restore our confidence in our present work. It helps us to regain a sense of perspective and proportion which we frequently lose in our efforts and without which no work is complete.'[2]

KEILIN asked the medical historian to record not only the achievements and successes of past times but also the unavoidable failures and disappointments which lie in the tortuous path of advance[3]. This advice does apply not only to the evaluation of more recent endeavors but equally to the interpretation of the experiments and doctrines of earlier periods. Medical history should not be written only as a record of achievements, since it becomes more instructive when we also follow the tortuous way of its errors.

1 VESALIUS, p. 643 (1543).
2 KEILIN, p. 3.
3 KEILIN, p. 1.

For this reason, I have attempted in this study not only to point out Galen's accomplishments but also to trace the erroneous trails of his thought. Evidently, Galen expressed many prejudices of his time and was at a disadvantage because of the primitive state of technology and basic science. Nevertheless, CLAUDE BERNARD's words apply equally to Galen's endeavor and to the students of modern science:

> 'In spite of our efforts, we are still very far from the absolute truth, and it is probable, especially in the biological sciences, that it will never be given to us to see it.'[4]

4 BERNARD, p. 54 (1878, reprint 1957).

BIBLIOGRAPHY

ARIENS-KAPPERS, C. M.; HUBER, G. C. and CROSBY, E. C.: *The comparative anatomy of the nervous system of vertebrates including man;* 2 vols. (only vol. 2 was used); (MacMillan, New York 1936).

ARISTOTLE: *Generation of animals;* Greek text with an English translation by A. L. PECK (Loeb Classical Library, Harvard University Press, Cambridge 1953).

— *On youth and old age;* Greek text with an English translation by W. S. HETT (Loeb Classical Library, Heinemann, London 1957).

— *Minor works: On colors;* Greek text with an English translation by W. S. HETT (Loeb Classical Library, Heinemann, London 1955).

— *On sense and sensible objects;* (for reference abbreviated: *De sensu*), Greek text with an English translation by W. S. HETT (Loeb Classical Library, Harvard University Press, Cambridge 1957).

— *De somnis et vigilia (On sleep and waking);* in same vol.

— *On the soul;* Greek text with an English translation by W. S. HETT (Loeb Classical Library, Heinemann, London 1957), in same vol.

— *Parva naturalia;* Greek text with an English translation by W. S. HETT (Loeb Classical Library, Harvard University Press, Cambridge 1957).

— *Physical problems;* (for reference abbreviated: *Problems*); Greek text with an English translation by W. S. HETT; 2 vols. (Loeb Classical Library, Harvard University Press 1961, 1965).

— *The works of Aristotle;* ed. by W. D. ROSS; vol. 2: *De generatione et corruptione* (The Clarendon Press, Oxford 1930).

— *The works of Aristotle;* ed. by W. D. ROSS; vol. 3: *Meteorologica; De anima; Parva naturalia; De spiritu* (Clarendon Press, Oxford 1951).

— *The works of Aristotle;* ed. by W. D. ROSS; vol. 4: *Historia animalium* (Clarendon Press, Oxford 1910).

— *Parts of animals;* Greek text with an English translation by A. L. PECK (Loeb Classical Library, Heinemann, London 1955).

— *Aristotle,* by W. D. ROSS (Methuen, London 1956).

ARNIM, J. VON: *Stoicorum veterum fragmenta*; collegit JOHANNES VON ARNIM; 4 vols. (Teubner, Stuttgart (1964), reprint of the edition of 1902.

ARNOLD, E. V.: *Roman Stoicism* (The Humanities Press, New York 1958).

BACON, R.: *Opus majus;* A translation by R. B. BURKE; 2 vols. (Russell and Russell, New York 1952).

BAILEY, C.: *The Greek Atomists and Epicurus* (Russell and Russell, New York 1964), reprint of edition of 1928.

BARTHOLINUS, C.: *Thomae Bartholini anatome ex omnium veterum recensiorumque observationibus* (ex officio Hackiana, Lugdun. Batav. 1673).

BAUR, L.: *Die philosophischen Werke des Robert Grosseteste, Bischof von Lincoln;* Beitr. Gesch. d. Philosoph. des Mittelalters, IX (1912).

BEARE, J. I.: *Greek theories of elementary cognition from Alcmaeon to Aristotle* (Oxford, Clarendon Press 1906), reprint.

BERNARD, C.: *An introduction to the study of experimental science (1878)*, transl. by H.C. GREENE (Dover, New York 1957).

BOYER, C. B.: *The rainbow, from myth to mathematics* (Yseloff, New York 1959).

BRETT, G. S.: *A history of psychology;* 3 vols. (Allen and Company, London 1912–1921).

— *History of psychology;* edited and abridged by R. S. PETERS (The MIT-Press, Cambridge, Mass. 1965).

BROCK, A. J.: *Galen on the natural faculties* (Loeb Classical Library, Heinemann, London 1952).

— *Greek medicine* (Dent & Sons, London 1929).

BROESICKE, G.: *Lehrbuch der normalen Anatomie* (Fischer, Berlin 1912).

CARR, D. E.: *Insects, animals and man;* The Atlantic Monthly, May 1967.

CASTIGLIONI, A.: *A history of medicine;* translated by E. B. KRUMBHAAR; 2nd ed. (Knopf, New York 1947).

CELSUS: *De medicina;* Latin text with an English translation by W. G. SPENCER; 3 vols. (Loeb Classical Library, Heinemann, London 1958).

CHERNISS, H.: *Galen's and Posidonius' theory of vision;* Amer. J. Philology *54:* 154–161 (1933).

CLARKE, E.: *Aristotle on the anatomy of the brain;* J. Hist. Med. and allied. Sci. *18:* 130–148 (1963).

— *Aristotelian concepts of the form and functions of the brain;* Bull. Hist. med. *37:* 1–14 (1963).

COHEN, M. R. and DRABKIN, I. E.: *A source book in Greek science* (Harvard University Press, Cambridge 1958).

CROMBIE, A. C.: *The study of the senses in Renaissance sciences;* Proc. Internat. Congress History of Sciences, pp. 92–114 (Hermann, Paris 1964).

— *Kepler, De modo visionis;* a translation from the Latin of *Ad Vitellionem Paralipomena*, ..., pp. 135–172 (Mélanges ALEXANDRE KOYRÉ).

— *Robert Grosseteste and the origins of experimental science 1100–1700* (The Clarendon Press, Oxford 1953).

— *The mechanistic hypothesis and the scientific study of vision; some optical ideas as a background to the invention of the microscope; in Historical Aspects of Microscopy;* ed. by S. BRADBURY and G. L. E. TURNER (Heffer & Sons, Cambridge 1967).

DAREMBERG, C.: *Œuvres anatomiques, physiologiques et médicales de Galien;* traduites (in French); 2 vols. (Baillière, Paris 1854). This translation of Galen which comprises some of his principal works will be referred to as 'DAREMBERG'.

— *Exposition de la connaissance de Galien sur l'anatomie, la physiologie et la pathologie du système nerveux,* thésis (Paris 1841) No. 222.

DESCARTES, R.: *Tractatus de homine;* Latin by DE LA FORGE (Elsevirius, Amsterdam 1677). See also the French text in the edition by C. ADAM and P. TANNERY (Cerf., Paris 1909: vol. 9).

DIELS, H. and KRANZ, W.: *Die Fragmente der Vorsokratiker;* 6th ed. by W. KRANZ; 2 vols. (Weidmann, Berlin 1951–1952).

DIEMERBROECK, I.: *Anatome corporis humani conscripta* (Huguetan, Lugduni 1679).

DIOGENES LAERTIUS: *Lives of eminent philosophers;* Greek text with an English translation by R. D. HICKS; 2 vols. (Loeb Classical Library, Heinemann, London 1959).

— more recent edition, see LONG, H. S.

DOWLING, J. E.: *Nightblindness;* Scientific American, *215:* 82 (1966).

DUCKWORTH, W. L. H.: *Galen on anatomical procedures, the later books;* English translation (University Press, Cambridge 1962).

DUKE-ELDER, S.: *System of ophthalmology;* ed. by S. DUKE-ELDER; vol. 1: *The eye in evolution* (Mosby, St. Louis 1958).

EPICURUS: see LONG, DIOGENES LAERTIUS, USENER.

EASTWOOD, B. S.: AVERROES' *view of the retina—A reappraisal,* J. Hist. Med. *24:* 77–82 (1969).

EUCLIDE: *L'optique et la catoptrique; œuvres traduites . . . avec une introduction et des notes;* par PAUL VER EECKE (Blanchard, Paris 1959).

EVANS, M. G.: *The physical philosophy of Aristotle* (University of New Mexico Press, Albuquerque 1964).

FREEMAN, K.: *The presocratic philosophers;* 3rd ed. (Blackwell, Oxford 1953).

GALEN: Interpretation: see SIEGEL.

— Translations: see BROCK, DAREMBERG, DUCKWORTH, MAY, SINGER, SIMON.

— *Claudii Galeni opera omnia;* ed. by D. C. G. KUEHN; 22 parts in 20 vols. (C. Cnobloch, Leipzig 1821–1833). A photoreprint has recently been made available of the entire edition. In all references this work will be referred to as 'KUEHN' followed by the number of volume and page.

GARRISON, F. H.: *An introduction to the history of medicine, 1929.* 4th edition; reprint (Saunders, Philadelphia 1963).

GOSS, CH. M.: *On anatomy of nerves by Galen of Permagon;* Amer. J. Anat. *118:* 327–335 (1966).

HALLER, A. VON: *Elementa physiologica;* 8 vols. (Grasset, Lausanne 1777–1778).

HARVEY, E. N.: *A history of luminescence* (American Philosophical Society, Philadelphia 1957).

HENSEL, H.: *Allgemeine Sinnesphysiologie,* Hautsinne, Geschmack, Geruch (Springer, Berlin 1966).

HIPPOCRATES: *Œuvres complètes;* trad. nouvelle avec text Grec, by E. LITTRÉ; 10 vols. (Baillière, Paris 1839–1861). Photoreprint now available.

HIRSCHBERG, J.: Geschichte d. Augenheilk.: vol. 12 of GRAEFE-SAEMISCH, Hdb. d. Augenheilk. (Engelmann, Leipzig 1899); also Berlin. Klin. Wschr. *56*: 635 (1919).

HORNE, R. A.: *Aristotelian chemistry;* Chymia *11:* 12–27 (1966).

HUBBARD, R. and KROPF, A.: *Molecular isomers in vision;* Scientific American *216:* 64–76 (1967).

ILBERG, J.: *Über die Schriftstellerei des Klaudios Galenos;* Rhein. Mus. N.F., vol. *44:* 207–239 (1889). This was continued in vols. *47:* 489–514 (1892); *51:* 165–196 (1896); *52:* 591–623 (1897).

JABLONSKI, W.: *Die Theorie des Sehens im griechischen Altertume bis auf Aristoteles;* Sudhoff's Arch. *23:* 306–333 (1930).

JOWETT, B.: see PLATO.

KEELE, K. D.: *Anatomies of pain* (Thomas, Springfield 1957).

KEILIN, D.: *History of cell respiration and cytochrome* (University Press, Cambridge 1967).

KIRK, G. S. and RAVEN, J. E.: *The presocratic philosophers, critical history with selection of texts* (University Press, Cambridge 1957).

KOELBING, H. M.: *Beobachtungen und Spekulation in der aristotelischen Sinnesphysiologie;* Dtsch. med. Wschr. *89:* 696–699 (1964).

KOLLESCH, J.: *Galen über das Riechorgan;* edited and with commentary (Akademie-Verlag, Berlin 1964).

KUEHN: Edition of Galen: See Galen.

LANDOIS, L. and ROSEMANN, R.: *Lehrbuch der Physiologie des Menschen;* 2 vols. (Urban und Schwarzenberg, Berlin 1919).

LEJEUNE, A.: *Euclide et Ptolémée: Deux stades de l'optique grecque* (Bibliothèque de L'Université, Louvain 1948).

— *L'optique de* CLAUDE PTOLÉMÉE: *dans la version latine d'après l'arabe;* édition critique par A. LEJEUNE (Publications Universitaires de Louvain 1956).

— *Recherches sur la catoptrique Grecque d'après les sources antiques et mediévales:* Acad. Royale de Belgique I classe lettres: Mémoires, tome 52, fasc. 2, Brussels 1957 (or 1954).

— *Les recherches de Ptolémée sur la vision binoculaire;* Janus *47:* 79–86 (1958).

LEONARDO DA VINCI: *The notebooks of...;* ed. by E. MACCURDY (Garden City Publishing Co., New York 1941–1942).

LEYACKER, J.: *Zur Entstehung der Lehre von den Hirnventrikeln als Sitz psychischer Vermögen;* Arch. Gesch. Med. *19:* 260 (1927).

LINDBERG, D. C.: ALHAZEN's *theory of vision and its reception in the West;* Isis *58:* 321–341 (1967).

LINKSZ, A.: *Physiology of the eye*; vol. 2: *Vision* (Grune and Stratton, New York 1952).

LISSMANN, H. W.: *The tropical fish Gymnarchus niloticus;* J. exp. Biol. *35:* 156–191 (1958).

LISSMANN, H. W. and MACHIN, K. E.: *The tropical fish Gymnarchus niloticus;* J. exp. Biol. *35:* 451–486 (1958).

LITTRÉ: see HIPPOCRATES.

LLOYD, G. E. R.: *Experiment in early Greek philosophy and medicine;* Proc. Cambridge Philol. Soc. *190:* 50–72 (1964).

LONG, H. S.: DIOGENES LAERTII *vita philosophorum;* 2 vols. (Clarendon Press, Oxford 1964).

LOWER, R.: *De catarrhis;* edited and translated by R. HUNTER and I. MACALPINE (Dawson, London 1963).

LUCRETIUS, T. CARUS: *De natura rerum, libri sex;* ed. by W. A. MERRILL (American Book Company, New York 1907).
— *On the nature of things,* literally translated in English prose, by J. S. WATSON (G. Bell and Sons, London 1886)

MACKENNA: see PLOTINUS
MAGNUS, H.: *Die Augenheilkunde der Alten* (Kern, Breslau 1901)[1].
MAY, M. T.: *Galen, On the usefulness of the parts of the body;* translated from the Greek with an introduction and commentary (Cornell University Press, Ithaca, New York 1968).—To my great regret this book was published after my own manuscript was already printed. Mrs. May's excellent translation should be used acc. to indication of book and chapter of Galen in my footnotes.
MAYER, C.L.: *Arabism, Egypt* and *Max Meyerhof;* Bull. Hist. med. *19:* 375–432 (1946).
METTLER, C.: *History of medicine;* ed. by F. A. METTLER (Blakiston, Philadelphia 1947).
MEYERHOF, O.: *Die Optic der Araber;* Z. opthalmologische Optic (three parts) *6:* 16, 42, 86 (1920).
MUELLER, I. VON: *Über Galen's Werk vom wissenschaftlichen Beweis;* Abh. der philol.-philosoph. Klasse der kgl. Bayer. Akad. der Wissenschaften, München II Abt. 20, pp. 403–478 (1897).
MUGLER, C.: *Sur l'histoire de quelques définitions de la géometrie grecque et les rapports entre la géométrie et l'optique;* Antiquité classique *26:* 331–345 (1957).

PANSIEN, P.: *Histoire des lunettes* (Malone, Paris 1901).
PENNINGTON, K. S.: *Advance in holography;* Scientific Amer. *218:* 40–44 (1968).
PLATO: *The dialogues of Plato;* translated into English with analyses and introductions by B. JOWETT: 4 vols.; 4th edition (Clarendon Press, Oxford, 1953).
— *Republic;* see Dialogues.
— *Timaeus;* Greek text with an English translation by R. G. BURY (Loeb Classical Library, Heinemann, London 1961).
PLOTINUS: *Enneades;* edited by R. VOLKMANN: 2 vols. (Teubner, Leipzig 1883–1884).
— *The Enneades;* translated by S. MACKENNA: 3rd edition (Pantheon Books, New York 1942, reprint 1966).
POLITZER, A.: *Geschichte der Ohrenheilkunde;* 2 vols. (Stuttgart, 1907–1913).
POLYAK, S.: *The vertebrate visual system;* ed. by H. KLUVER (University of Chicago Prcss, Chicago 1957).
PTOLÉMÉE: see LEJEUNE.

RONCHI, V.: *Histoire de la lumière;* translated from the Italian and revised by E. ROSEN (Librairie Armand, Paris 1957).

SAMBURSKI, S.: *Physics of the Stoics* (Routledge and Kegan Paul, London 1959).
— *The physical world of the Greeks;* translated from the Hebrew by M. DAGUT (Routledge and Kegan Paul, London 1956).
— *The physical world of late antiquity* (Routledge and Kegan Paul, London 1962).

[1] His frequent misinterpretations of Galen could not be discussed in my analysis.

SARTON, G.: *An introduction to the history of science;* vol. 1 (William and Wilkins, Baltimore 1953).
— *Galen of Pergamon* (Univ. of Kansas Press, Lawrence 1954).
SCHOENE, R.: DAMIANOS' *Schrift über die Optik,* Berlin, 1897; (German and Greek text).
SHASTID, TH. H.: *History of ophthalmology;* in *Dictionary of ophthalmology;* ed. by C. A. WOOD; vol. 11, pp. 8525–8904 (Cleveland Press, Chicago 1911).
SHUTE, C.: *The psychology of Aristotle, an analysis of the living being* (Columbia University Press, New York 1941).
SIEGEL, R. E.: *Theories of vision and color perception of Empedocles and Democritus; some similarities to the modern approach,* Bull. Hist. med. *33:* 145–159 (1959).
— *The paradoxes of Zeno; some similarities between ancient Greek and modern thought;* Janus *48:* 24–47 (1959).
— HIPPOCRATES' *description of metabolic diseases in relation to modern concepts;* Bull. Hist. med. *34:* 355–364 (1960).
— *Galen's experiments and observations on pulmonary blood flow and respiration;* Am. J. Cardiol. *10:* 738–745 (1962).
— *The influence of Galen's doctrine of pulmonary blood flow on the development of modern concepts of circulation;* Sudhoffs Arch. *46:* 311–332 (1962).
— *Clinical observations in* HIPPOCRATES, *an essay on the evolution of the diagnostic art;* J. Mount Sinai Hospital *31:* 285–302 (1964).
— *Galen's system of medicine and physiology, an analysis of his doctrines on blood flow, respiration, humors and internal diseases;* 419 pages (Karger, Basel 1968).
SIMON, M.: *Sieben Bücher der Anatomie des Galen;* vol. 2 (Hinrich, Leipzig 1906).
SINGER, C.: *Galen on anatomical procedures;* translated with introduction and notes (Oxford University Press, London 1956).
SISSON, S. and GROSSMAN, J. D.: *The anatomy of domestic animals* (Saunders, Philadelphia, 4th ed., 1956).
SOLMSEN, F.: *'Aisthesis' in Aristotelian and Epicurean thought.* Medelingen der Koninkl. Nederlandse Akademie van Wetenschappen, Nieuwe Reeks, Deel 24, No. 8, pp. 239–262 (Amsterdam 1961).
— *Cleanthes or Posidonius? The basis of Stoic physics;* Medelingen der Koninkl. Nederlandse Akademie van Wetenschappen, Nieuwe Reeks, Deel 24, No. 9, pp. 263–289 (Amsterdam 1961).
SOURY, J.: *Le système nerveux central, structure et fonctions; histoire critique des théories et des doctrines;* 2 vols. (Impr. Nationale, Paris 1899).
STERNBACH, R. A.: *Pain, a psycho-physiological analysis* (Academy Press, New York 1968).
STOICS: see VON ARNIM.
STARLING'S *Principles of human physiology;* 7th ed. by C. L. EVANS (Churchill, London 1936).
STRATTON, G. M.: *Theophrastus and the Greek physiological psychology before Aristotle* (Allen and Unwin, London 1917).

THEOPHRASTUS, see STRATTON.

USENER, H.: *Epicurea;* L'Herma di Breitschneider, Rome 1963 (photoreprint).

Ver Eecke, P.: see Euclide.
Vesalius, A.: *De humani corporis fabrica,* 1543 (reprint, Bruxelles 1964).
Von Arnim: see Arnim, J.
Von Mueller: see Mueller, I. von.

Walzer, R.: *Galen on medical experience* (Oxford University Press 1946).
Werner, H.: *Die galenische Otologie;* Diss. (Zurich 1925).
White, J. C. and Sweet, W. H.: *Pain, its mechanism and neuro-surgical control* (C. C. Thomas, Springfield, Ill. 1955).
Wright, S.: *Applied physiology* (Oxford Univ. Press, London 1945).

INDEX OF NAMES

INDEX OF SUBJECTS